THE
JOURNEY
TO
RECOVERY

THE JOURNEY TO RECOVERY

A Complete Guide to Cancer Chemotherapy

Margot Joan Fromer

Adams Media Corporation
Holbrook, Massachusetts

Published by
Adams Media Corporation
260 Center Street, Holbrook, MA 02343. U.S.A.
www.adamsmedia.com

ISBN: 1-58062-446-4

Printed in Canada.

J   I   H   G   F   E   D   C   B   A

Cataloging-in-Publication data available
upon request from the publisher.

This publication is designed to provide accurate and authoritative information with regard to the subject matter covered. It is sold with the understanding that the publisher is not engaged in rendering legal, accounting, or
other professional advice. If legal advice or other expert assistance is required,
the services of a competent professional person should be sought.
—From a *Declaration of Principles* jointly adopted
by a Committee of the American Bar Association and a Committee of
Publishers and Associations

Many of the designations used by manufacturers and sellers to distinguish
their products are claimed as trademarks. Where those designations appear in
this book and Adams Media was aware of a trademark claim, the designations have been printed in initial capital letters.

This book is available at quantity discounts for bulk purchases.
For information, call 1-800-872-5627.

Dedicated to the memory of
Beatrice Neuman Fromer

Birth is a beginning
And death a destination.
And life is a journey:
From childhood to maturity
And youth to age;
From innocence to awareness
And ignorance to knowing;
From foolishness to discretion
    And then, perhaps, to wisdom;
From weakness to strength
Or strength to weakness—
    And often, back again;
From health to sickness
    And back, we pray, to health again;
From offense to forgiveness,
From loneliness to love,
From joy to gratitude,
From pain to compassion,
And grief to understanding—
    From fear to faith;
From defeat to defeat to defeat—
Until, looking backward or ahead,
We see that victory lies
Not at some high place along the way,
But in having made the journey, stage by stage,
    A sacred pilgrimage.
Birth is a beginning
And death a destination.
And life is a journey,
A sacred pilgrimage—
    To life everlasting.

—*Gates of Repentance*
Central Conference of American Rabbis, 1996

Contents

Foreword

The word *cancer* is such a simple one, yet it wields tremendous power capable of instilling fear, despair, and a sense of hopelessness. I remember the first time I actually heard the word *cancer*. I was a second-year medical student busily doing what medical students do: trying to learn all I could about disease and how to cure it. Like most of my classmates, I thought I knew about human nature and about life in general, and I did not think I had to learn much about human behavior. Medical facts were the important things. How does one diagnose heart failure? What is the proper treatment for pneumonia? This is the information my colleagues and I sought to learn.

Even though I was only in my mid-twenties, I felt I knew a lot about the way humans react to serious illnesses. After all, I had experienced illness in my own family with the death of my grandparents, as well as my father's chronic illness that completely debilitated him. All these problems were taken in stride as part of living and dying. I felt I was compassionate and understanding of my patients' needs because of my own experiences. Then I received a call from my father informing me that my mother, who had been ill but was seemingly getting better, had cancer. There was that word again—*cancer*.

I suddenly realized I knew very little about the disease. All I knew was that it was generally bad and that my mother was not yet fifty years old. I knew even less about what I could do to help her. I felt strangely ignorant and lost. What should I do? What did I know?

Then she died.

I remember my family's sense of despair and helplessness as we watched this woman of great warmth and compassion quickly fade away. We asked many questions during the course of her illness but received few answers. Our family doctor was an immensely compassionate person but gave us little useful information. There were no how-to books available on the subject of terminal illness and cancer care. We were completely lost.

Twenty-five years later, I see this scenario repeated nearly every day of my professional life. As an oncologist, I am often transported back to that day when I learned that my mother had cancer, and I remember all too well the fear, uncertainty, and ignorance my family and I felt. Accurate information is essential when confronting any illness, but it is especially important when dealing with a life-threatening disease like cancer.

Margot Fromer has written a wonderful manual for those of us who have cancer. (I too have had cancer and experienced all the fear and anxiety that accompanies the disease.) Family members will find answers to many of their questions about their loved one's illness. Fromer takes us through the basics of cancer biology in a clear and lucid manner. She explains the rationale behind the therapies oncologists use to treat cancer, and she provides us with the why and how of treatment. Management of common side effects is succinctly described. She provides very practical information about clinical trials—what they are and whether one should get involved. Fromer also provides pragmatic advice on how to pay for therapy, an increasingly challenging facet of cancer in this world of limited resources.

In short, Fromer's book should be enormously helpful to anyone with a diagnosis of cancer or a family member or friend seeking to understand more about this collection of diseases. I only wish such a book had been available 25 years ago when my family and I were faced with this diagnosis in my mother. She too would have found Fromer's book extremely useful in her struggle against a very difficult disease.

David H. Johnson, M.D.
Director, Division of Hematology & Oncology
Vanderbilt-Ingram Cancer Center
Vanderbilt University Medical School

Member, Board of Directors
American Society of Clinical Oncology

Introduction

*A*lthough you may be terribly frightened of even the thought of cancer, it is no longer an automatic death sentence. This is said so often, in fact, that it sounds like a cliché. But the truth is that it *is* a fact: more people than ever survive cancer and go on to live happy, normal, and productive lives. Almost all of these increases in survival and good health are the result of chemotherapy.

Surgery and radiation, the other two major types of cancer treatment, still have a strong place in cancer therapeutics, and they will be discussed briefly in this book. However, it is *chemotherapy* (the use of drugs and biologics to fight the disease) that has caused cancer to evolve from a hopeless and always fatal group of diseases to what in many cases is a chronic disease that can be controlled and often cured entirely

In fact, about half of all diagnosed cancers are cured (up from 39 percent in 1973 to 56 percent today), and the National Cancer Institute (NCI) estimates that more than 8 million Americans alive today have had cancer. More than 300,000 Americans each year can say, "I *had* cancer, but I don't now." It is highly likely that if you were diagnosed early and began treatment right away, you too will regain your health.

This is not to say that your cancer is definitely curable, because some types of the disease have a much higher cure rate than others, and factors other than the type and amount of treatment affect whether you will survive it. But even if cancer cannot be definitively cured, chemotherapy has greatly extended survival time and has given people a much improved quality of life for the time remaining to them. As a result of chemotherapy, many cancer patients who still have the disease live quite normal lives. All of this is the result of modern chemotherapy.

Chemotherapy, sometimes accompanied by surgery, radiation, or hormone therapy, has become the first line of attack in treating cancer, and often it is the *only* possible line of attack. Your treatment, of course, will be designed specifically for you. It will depend on the type of cancer you have, when it was diagnosed, whether and where it has spread, and many other factors. And your *oncologist* (a physician who specializes in treating cancer) will explain why he or she is recommending this or that treatment. If you don't receive an explanation, ask for one; we'll discuss this more later in the book.

Although the course of chemotherapy can be rocky at times—in fact, most people say it is no fun at all—in almost every single instance, if your doctor recommends chemotherapy, you will benefit from it in several ways. It is a temporary inconvenience that will produce long-term health benefits.

After you have been diagnosed with cancer, and probably even before the shock of hearing your doctor say the dread word has worn off and you have become accustomed to being a cancer patient, treatment will begin. It is axiomatic that the earlier the disease is diagnosed and treatment begun, the better the chance of survival and ultimate cure. Therefore, if chemotherapy is the most appropriate treatment for you, it will begin immediately—and it will be the most aggressive treatment your doctor thinks will be effective and safe. Using the word *aggressive* in the same sentence as *medical treatment*— on *your* body—might make you feel as though you want to run as fast as you can in the opposite direction. But don't. Stay and listen to what your doctor is telling you and why the drugs he or she is suggesting are the most appropriate for you at that particular time.

As you read further into this book, you will learn why certain drugs are used in certain diseases, but the short answer to why chemotherapy has to be aggressive is this: cancer is an aggressive disease. In fact, it is a malevolent disease that, if left to its own devices, will consume you. It will kill you. Therefore, it has to be fought on its own terms. The cancer cells must be killed—and that's pretty aggressive.

You will be tossed into a world that you probably never knew existed—one populated by strangers who speak a language that not only sounds foreign (it is—to you) but seems designed to keep you in the dark about your own disease and treatment. In the beginning, you will be shunted from specialist to specialist, from department to department in the hospital, from laboratory to laboratory. You'll feel alone, scared, and angry. This is normal. The fact that it happens to everyone who has ever had cancer won't be a comfort—at least at first.

What *can* be a comfort and a help, however, is knowing and understanding what is happening to you. That is what this book is for. There are upwards of 120 drugs and other agents used alone, or more commonly in combination, to treat cancer. *The Journey to Recovery: A Complete Guide to Cancer Chemotherapy* will list and describe each one of them, as well as specify for which cancers they are usually used. The book serves as a guide to what cancer is, how chemotherapeutic agents work, and what the side effects are—and how to cope with and minimize them. It also explains biological agents, investigational drugs (those that are still being tested in humans), and clinical trials—as well as nontraditional cancer therapy that you should beware of. The heart of the book, however, is the drugs themselves: what they are, how they are classified, how they act on both malignant and normal cells, and which cancers they are used to treat.

Although the idea of treating cancer with chemicals and naturally occurring substances has been around since the time of Hippocrates in ancient Greece, the practice of chemotherapy didn't begin until World War II—and then it was a crude and haphazard business. Nitrogen mustard was the first chemical approved by the Food and Drug Administration to treat cancer, and it remained the only drug in the cancer armamentarium for the next 20 years.

Research began in earnest in the 1950s, and from the mid-1960s, when President Nixon declared war on cancer, research on cancer drugs, as well as on the nature of the disease itself, has been progressing steadily and rapidly. Along with chemotherapy itself have come drugs to minimize side effects. Today, some cancers can be cured entirely through the use of chemotherapy: testicular cancer, Hodgkin's disease, some non-Hodgkin's lymphomas, some leukemias, and even some types of ovarian cancer.

Not only is there a wide variety of chemotherapeutic agents available to treat cancer, but they are more sophisticated than ever. That is, they are designed to target specific cells while leaving others alone. This makes them more potent in attacking the cancer while producing fewer and more manageable side effects. For instance, not everyone loses their hair, and most people don't lose a great deal of weight.

Because the treatment of cancer, particularly with drugs, is always changing, and because new drugs are being discovered, tested, and approved at an ever-increasing rate, this or any book cannot and should not serve as the final or definitive word on the course of treatment you should pursue. Only you and your physician can make that decision.

Cancer chemotherapy is a journey. From a frightening departure point, through some challenging terrain, most people arrive at a destination of renewed health and strength. Use *The Journey to Recovery: A Complete Guide to Cancer Chemotherapy* as a source of information, to answer questions you might have forgotten to ask your doctor, and to help your friends and family better understand what you are going through. Use it in good health.

Chapter One

The Biology of Cancer

The Many Forms of Cancer:
What It Is, Why It Occurs, and How It Is Detected

Demography of Cancer

Although cancer can and does strike anyone of any race, of any gender, and at any age, it does have demographic characteristics that make it, if not predictive of incidence and occurrence, at least indicative of some general patterns.

Age

In general, the older you are, the more likely you are to fall victim to cancer. In fact, age is one of the most significant factors for cancer. The median age at diagnosis is 67, and more than two-thirds of all cancer deaths occur after age 65. Several reasons account for the relationship of aging to cancer: immune function diminishes as the body ages; the body's ability to repair damaged cells declines with time, and damage may be cumulative and act as a causative factor in the development of malignancies; and the longer one lives, the longer one has been exposed to various carcinogens (cancer-causing agents), and the more time slow-growing cancers have to develop.

Gender

Cancer is "sexist." That is, overall, men run a greater risk of the disease. More than 125,000 more men than women develop cancer every year, probably due to differences in lifestyle, especially greater exposure to chemical carcinogens in the workplace.

Except for skin cancer, prostate and breast cancers are the most common malignancies in men and women, the second largest cause

I

of cancer deaths for each gender—and among the most rapidly increasing cancers in the United States. Lung cancer, which used to kill far more men than women, is now much more gender neutral. This is because the incidence of lung cancer in men began to drop in the mid-1980s, just as it began to increase dramatically in women, and in 1987, it surpassed breast cancer as the leading cancer killer of women. This is due almost entirely to smoking patterns among Americans.

Socioeconomic Factors

Poverty, lack of education, and membership in certain racial minorities (especially blacks) increase the risk of developing—and dying from—cancer in the United States. Black men have the highest rate of cancer of any population group in this country, and black men and women have a much lower five-year survival rate than do white men and women. Native Hawaiians, and people of Japanese, Chinese, Hispanic, and Filipino descent, all have higher rates of cancer than do whites, but American Indians have the lowest rate of all U.S. population groups. A number of factors contribute to these differences:

> Genetic susceptibility
> Differences in lifestyle and nutritional habits
> Alcohol and tobacco use, which correlates with income and education
> Differences in access to screening programs
> Financial resources and purchase of health insurance
> Childbearing patterns

Family

Some cancers are definitely hereditary, such as retinoblastoma, a cancer of the retina in the eye; Siple's syndrome, which causes thyroid cancer; and the Li-Fraumeni syndrome, which causes various malignancies. Others, such as breast cancer and certain colon cancers, have a clear tendency to run in families.

What Makes a Cell Malignant

When one says "I have cancer," or "My Aunt Sylvia just found out she has cancer," the statement is not entirely accurate. Cancer is not a single disease but rather one of about 200 conditions in which body cells behave in certain abnormal ways. These conditions have basic things in common, but they also differ in significant ways.

Although there is no single definition that accurately defines all types of malignancies, in general, *cancer* is the word used for abnormal growth of cells. The two major characteristics of this abnormal growth are out-of-control multiplication, and change in the cells' structure, function (shape and activity), and location. When these two conditions occur at the same time, the cells are said to be *malignant*—or cancerous.

Other abnormal cell growths are not cancer. They are known as *lesions* or *neoplasms* and rarely become malignant. Some groups of abnormal cells, such as polyps, are called *dysplasia*, and they are generally considered premalignant. Depending on where they are, they are either removed or carefully watched. *Hyperplasia* is an increase in the number of cells in a particular place, such as in response to a cut or surgical wound. This is entirely normal; as soon as healing is complete, the number of cells returns to normal.

When physicians talk about cancer, they generally refer not so much to the disease itself but to the *tumor*, the central malignant source of the disease. In cancer diagnosis and treatment, the size and condition of the tumor is all important—how big it is at the time of diagnosis, how much of it was removed during surgery, and how quickly and completely it shrinks as a result of chemotherapy.

Tumors

A tumor is a mass of cells without a biological purpose. (By the way, a word ending in *–oma* usually refers to a tumor.) Every single cell in your body has a definite purpose, which may be simple or complex, but the purpose is always part of the grand design to maintain life and health. For instance, skin cells form the outer covering of the body; cells of the small intestine are responsible for absorption of the nutrients that pass through the digestive system; liver cells perform a wide variety of chemical functions having to do with metabolism and release of enzymes; and brain cells regulate all body functions and make you who you are. In contrast, cancer cells do not maintain life and health, and they destroy healthy tissue.

Cancer begins with a small number of abnormal cells—sometimes only one cell— which rapidly multiply. Different cancers grow at different rates; some take years before they are detectable and cause symptoms. The multiplying cells eventually form a malignant tumor (a clump of cancer cells). The tumor may stay in one place (cancer *in situ*) for varying lengths of time, but eventually it *metastasizes* (spreads) to other parts of the body. The part of the body in which the cancer first develops is called the *primary site*, and no matter where it spreads, it is always referred to by its primary name. For instance a woman with breast cancer whose disease has spread to her brain, chest, or ovary is always referred to as having breast cancer even though treatment is directed toward other body parts. It is possible, though rare, to have more than one primary cancer at the same time. It is also possible to have cancer of an unknown primary site.

Cancer cells have a number of characteristics. They do not look like normal cells, although many have a similar appearance. They may be a different size and shape, have larger or smaller nuclei, and may not fit together in a normal pattern. Neither do they function in the way in which they were designed. In fact, cancer cells have no normal function.

Cancer cells grow at a faster than normal rate, and they often appear immature because they divide and reproduce before they reach full maturity. They are likely to mutate again, and they have a higher than usual tendency to break off from their clusters and travel to other parts of the body. Many of these misplaced cells are destroyed by the immune system, but if they survive and attach themselves to new tissue, the cancer spreads.

Not all tumors are malignant. Everyone at some time in their lives has one or more benign tumors, such as moles, wens, and lumps of fatty tissue under the skin. They are not harmful, will not spread, and should be left alone unless you want them removed for cosmetic reasons. A malignant tumor, on the other hand, has no wall of tissue around it, nor does it have clear-cut borders. Rather, it is irregularly shaped and sends out a network of new blood vessels through which cells break off from the original tumor and spread to the rest of the body via the general circulation. (This is called *angiogenesis* and will be discussed in Chapter 4.) Other characteristics of tumors include (1) a silent period, which usually occurs when the cancer first develops, when there is minimal or no growth and no symptoms; (2) organs of affinity, that is, the organs to which the original malignant cells have a tendency to spread, such as from breast to brain, bone, or ovary; and (3) a specific growth rate.

You may have heard the term *tumor marker*, which has received a good deal of coverage in the press recently. A tumor marker is a chemical substance, many of which are produced by the tumor itself, found in increased amounts in the body fluids of people with cancer. Each one of these chemicals is specific for a certain type of cancer. Therefore, a blood test that reveals a particular tumor marker may indicate a particular type of cancer. The word *may* is important because tumor marker tests are often inaccurate, and false positive results are common; thus tumor markers do not constitute a definitive diagnosis of cancer. Tumor markers also are used to monitor the progress of treatment and to detect a recurrence of the cancer after the disease is cured or has gone into long-term remission.

Types of Tumors

One of the ways in which malignant tumors differ from one another is the body tissue in which they develop and grow. There are several types of tumors.

Carcinomas, by far the most common type , develop in epithelial tissue that covers the surface of or forms the lining of organs and passageways. Most carcinomas form in organs that secrete a substance. For example, lungs secrete mucous; breasts secrete milk; and the pancreas, stomach, and intestines secrete digestive juices. An *adenocarcinoma* arises in the cells' lining or on the surface of an organ or gland in any part of the body; *squamous cell* carcinoma originates in the skin. *Melanoma* also begins in the skin. Carcinoma in situ refers to a cancer that remains confined to its site of origin. This is the most easily curable by surgery alone. Common carcinomas include the following:

> ➤ *Breast cancer*, the second most frequent cancer in women in the United States (after skin cancers), accounts for one-third of all cancer diagnoses. Estrogen probably plays a significant causative role in breast cancer, and about 5 percent of all cases of the disease are hereditary (two breast cancer genes have now been identified). Increasing age also is a major risk factor. The single most important factor in successfully treating breast cancer is early detection—by annual mammography for all women over the age of 40.

➤ *Thyroid cancer* is very uncommon, and it is usually so slow-growing that people die of other causes before their cancer is detectable. Radiation to the head and neck, especially in childhood, may be one of the causative factors in thyroid cancer, and about 20 percent of thyroid cancers are inherited.

➤ *Pancreatic cancer* is a highly deadly form of the disease because there are no screening tests to detect it, and it is asymptomatic until far advanced—and even then, the symptoms are very vague. Pancreatic cancer spreads to the stomach, upper small intestine, and the surrounding lymph nodes.

➤ *Squamous cell carcinoma* occurs in the surface cells of the lining of the vagina (and other organs with similar types of mucous membrane such as the rectum), usually in the upper third of the organ near the cervix. Most vaginal cancers are not primary; they have metastasized from another primary site—usually the colon, uterus, or stomach. There is a strong association between squamous cell carcinomas of the vagina and rectum and human papilloma viruses, which are sexually transmitted. Squamous cell carcinomas also are found in the cervix, esophagus (which is due almost entirely to cigarette smoking), non-small cell lung cancer, bladder cancer, oral and nasal carcinomas, and skin cancer.

➤ *Basal cell carcinoma*, one type of skin cancer (the others are squamous cell and melanoma), occurs most often on the head and neck, particularly the nose, eyelids, and cheeks. These cancers grow slowly and rarely metastasize. Skin cancer in general has a very high cure rate (100 percent if it is diagnosed before it spreads), and it is one of the most preventable because almost all cases are caused by overexposure to sunlight.

➤ *Adenocarcinoma* develops in glandular tissues such as the vagina, cervix, uterus, esophagus, stomach (risk factors for which include prolonged exposure to foods containing nitrates, as well as prior infection with *Helicobacter pylori*, the bacterium that causes ulcers), colon, rectum, gallbladder, bile ducts, lung, kidney, bladder, salivary glands, pharynx, and larynx.

➤ *Ovarian carcinoma* has the highest mortality rate of all cancers in women because it is almost completely asymptomatic until it has advanced and metastasized. It tends to be familial in nature, although direct causes are unknown. The vast majority of ovarian cancers start in the epithelium, the covering of the ovary, and most of the rest arise from the cells that produce ova (eggs).

Sarcomas develop in bone or soft tissue that supports bone (muscles, nerves, cartilage, tendons, fat, and the like). Since these tissues are found all over the body, a sarcoma can arise anywhere. Common sarcomas include the following:

- *Osteosarcoma*, bone cancer, is most common in adolescents and young adults, and usually begins in the arms and legs. Bone cancer, as well as other sarcomas, metastasizes rapidly and has a special affinity for the lungs.
- *Chondrosarcoma*, another bone cancer, arises in the cartilage of the pelvis, thigh, and shoulder.
- *Ewing's sarcoma*, the rarest type of bone cancer, begins in the pelvis or lower legs.
- *Soft tissue sarcomas* are named for the tissues in which they originate. Periosteal sarcoma begins in the fibrous tissue that covers bones; angiosarcoma begins in blood vessels; and rhabdomyosarcoma arises in skeletal muscle. The tumors grow outward from their point of origin and encroach on adjacent tissue, including nerves, which usually makes sarcomas extremely painful as they grow. If the tumor invades blood vessels, circulatory problems ensue; if it grows into the bowel or urinary tract, obstructions occur.
- *Kaposi's sarcoma*, formerly an extremely rare cancer, arises from blood vessels and is one of the defining signs of AIDS. It is almost certainly linked to viral infection and to compromise of the immune system. Internal and external lesions associated with Kaposi's sarcoma are disseminated widely around the body, and the disease spreads rapidly.

Lymphomas, *lymphosarcomas*, and *leukemias*, also called liquid tumors, develop in the lymph glands or the blood-forming cells of the bone marrow. Liquid tumors include the following:

➤ *Acute leukemia* is cancer of the bone marrow and lymphatic system. Leukemia is the most common type of childhood cancer, but it affects nine times as many adults as children. In acute leukemia, immature blood cells proliferate rapidly and overtake mature white blood cells and in time interfere with the normal function of almost all tissues and organs. In addition, the growth of abnormal white cells prevents production of red cells and platelets, thus leaving the person with leukemia at great risk of infection and hemorrhage. The two major subgroups of acute leukemia are *myeloid* and *lymphoid*, named for the type of white blood cells in which they arise.

➤ *Chronic leukemia*, the most common form of the disease in adults, affects blood cells at a later stage of development. They appear mature but do not function normally. Chronic leukemia may have a genetic component, and there are probably links between the disease and environmental risk factors such as exposure to benzene or high doses of radiation. The two major types of chronic leukemia are *myeloid* and *lymphoid*.

➤ *Hodgkin's disease* affects the lymphatic system and generally strikes young adults. It is highly curable (60 to 70 percent survive 10 years or more), and may be causally related to the Epstein-Barr virus, which is also the cause of mononucleosis. In Hodgkin's disease, abnormal lymph cells (these are called Reed-Sternberg cells and are unique to Hodgkin's disease) proliferate much more rapidly than normal ones, thus interfering with the body's ability to fight infection.

➤ *Non-Hodgkin's lymphoma*, a group of diseases that is increasing in the United States, is probably caused by viruses, particularly Epstein-Barr, and/or genetic defects. It is particularly common in people who are infected by the human immunodeficiency virus (HIV) and those who have received immunosuppressive drugs following organ transplants. Non-Hodgkin's lymphomas, of which there are several types, are very similar to Hodgkin's save for the presence of Reed-Sternberg cells. Lymphomas are characterized as aggressive when tumor cells grow rapidly, and they are considered indolent when the cells grow more slowly. The incidence of aggressive and indolent disease is roughly equal.

➤ *Multiple myeloma* is the most common of a group of cancers called *plasma cell neoplasms*. Plasma cells are one of the B-lymphocytes that normally do not multiply (see Chapter 3 for a discussion of blood components). But in the presence of a plasma cell neoplasm, they proliferate, develop abnormally, and produce an overabundance of antibodies called immunoglobulins. The abnormal cells are called myeloma cells. Multiple myeloma is a rare cancer (as are all plasma cell neoplasms), but it is on the increase in the United States, possibly because of exposure to radiation and/or environmental chemicals.

Cancers of nervous tissue are named after the cells they affect. The most common cancer of the central nervous system (which comprises the brain and spinal cord) is *primary brain cancer*, prevalent in children and young adults as well as in people over age 50, in whom the incidence is increasing. Because brain tumors arise in an enclosed space, there is almost no room for them to grow. For this reason, they are symptomatic in early stages, whereas many other cancers don't make themselves known clinically until they are far advanced. The two major types of primary brain tumors are *gliomas* and *nongliomas*. Gliomas arise from glial cells and include *astrocytoma* (the most common and one of the most deadly), *brain stem glioma*, and mixed tumors that involve more than one type of glial cell. Examples of nonglial tumors include *acoustic neurinoma* (arising from the acoustic nerve), *meningioma* (arising from the meninges, the covering of the brain), and *craniopharyngioma* (arising from a structure near the pituitary gland).

Neuroblastoma is another type of nervous tissue cancer, this time in the sympathetic nervous system, which regulates the body's involuntary functions such as heart rate, digestion, and respiration. A neuroblastoma can occur anywhere in the body but most commonly in the abdomen.

Cancer also can arise from an unknown primary source. It is called *occult primary* or *carcinoma of unknown primary (CUP)*, and it is exactly what it sounds like—a mystery. CUP is usually asymptomatic until it has metastasized, and then the symptoms arise from the metastatic sites and the cells are typical of metastatic cancer. The two most common sites where CUP is detected are the lung and the pancreas.

Causes of Cancer

There is no one single cause of cancer, although in the United States, cigarette smoking is the most important single identified cause of the disease. It is responsible for more than 100,000 deaths a year from lung cancer alone, as well as additional cases and deaths of cancer of the mouth, throat, esophagus, pancreas, bladder, and pleura (lining of the lungs).

The Immune System

One theory of the causation of cancer holds that the immune system has broken down in some way, which results in a condition called *immunosuppression* or *immunodeficiency*. To explain further: everyone produces a number of cancerous or mutant cells, and under normal circumstances, they are perceived as "foreign invaders" and destroyed by the immune system. In people who develop cancer, some of these cells, for a variety of biochemical reasons, are not recognized and attacked by the immune system. Thus, they continue to grow unchecked.

Genetics

Scientists have recently discovered that some normal genes are transformed into genes that promote the development of cancer. These are called *oncogenes* (from the Greek *onkos*, meaning mass or tumor). In every cell of the human body there are 50,000 to 100,000 genes, of which only about 100 or so regulate cell growth or division. These are the ones that have the potential to mutate into oncogenes.

Mutation is a two-step process: *initiation* and *promotion*. The cell DNA (deoxyribonucleic acid) itself must change, which in turn transforms the normal cell into a tumor cell. But what causes the DNA to change in the first place? There are several theories. First, viruses may insert their own DNA into a cell's DNA. Second, a "carcinogenic bullet" or a number of these bullets (known as the "multiple hit" theory) can hit a cell in just the right spot to make it turn cancerous. These bullets or hits come from chemicals or foreign substances that cause cancer (carcinogens), such as tobacco and tobacco smoke, x-rays and other types of radiation, hormones, excessive exposure to sunlight, industrial or chemical agents (including benzene, asbestos, vinyl chloride, and arsenic), and excesses or deficiencies of certain nutrients. Third, carcinogenic promoters may accelerate the growth of abnormal cells. These promoters include alcohol, stress, and heredity.

Infectious Agents

Various infectious agents are known or suspected to be implicated as causative factors in malignancy. Proving a cause-and-effect relationship has been difficult, however, because of the long incubation period of many infectious diseases as well as the variety of other factors needed to turn an infection into a cancer. Three types of infectious agents have been implicated: bacteria, fungi, and viruses.

Bacteria

The best documented relationship between bacterial infection and malignancy is between *Helicobacter pylori* (*H. pylori*) and stomach cancer. This is the same bacterium that causes stomach and duodenal ulcers. *H. pylori* changes the cellular structure of the stomach lining, which results in chronic inflammation and permanently reduced acid. After 15 years of infection with *H. pylori*, the risk of cancer is 8 times what it is in non-infected people, and in fact, *H. pylori* is probably responsible for about 60 percent of all stomach cancers.

Other common bacteria implicated in cancer causation are those found in the colon, such as the *Bacteroides* species, which mutate bile salts into carcinogens.

Fungi

Molds and fungi in certain pickled vegetables produce carcinogens called nitrosamines, which may cause cancer in and of themselves and may also enhance other carcinogens. These molds and fungi include *Fusarium, Alternaria, Geotrichum, Aspergillis, Penicillium*, and others.

Flukes and bloodflukes have been linked to cancer in mechanisms similar to those caused by chronic bacterial infection. They include *Opisthorchis viverrini, Clonorchis sinesnsis, Fasciola hepatica*, and *Schistosoma haematobium*.

Viruses

Viruses are by far the most common infectious agents implicated in cancer causation. The mechanisms by which these smallest of unicellular creatures cause malignancy are being widely studied, and a good deal is now understood. In general, a virus penetrates a cell (or more likely, many cells) and alters the DNA, which in turn leads to a loss of control of cellular reproduction.

Cat owners have long been familiar with the risk of feline leukemia virus (FeLV), which is highly contagious. FeLV is a chronic ongogenic virus associated with both immunosuppression and malignancy. It has been used as an animal model for human immunosuppressive virus (HIV), the causative agent in AIDS. HIV also has been linked to non-Hodgkin's lymphoma, Hodgkin's disease, cervical and anorectal carcinomas, Kaposi's sarcoma, and cancers of the mouth.

Other connections between viruses and cancer include the following:

> Epstein-Barr virus (EBV) is a causative factor in non-Hodgkin's lymphomas, especially in people already suffering from AIDS. EBV also has been implicated in Hodgkin's disease, salivary gland carcinoma, urogenital cancer, lymphoblastic lymphoma, T-cell lymphoma, leiomyosarcoma, and Burkitt's lymphoma.

> Co-infection with human papilloma virus (HPV) and HIV creates a predisposition to anogenital carcinomas. HPV also is associated with skin cancers in kidney transplant patients, esophageal carcinoma, penile cancer, and anal cancer.

> Human T-cell leukemic viruses (HTLV-I and HTLV-II), which also are retroviruses, have strong oncogenic properties and have been closely associated with adult T-cell leukemia.

> Hepatitis B virus (HBV) affects about 200 million people around the world; it is associated with liver cancer, very often preceded by cirrhosis of the liver.

> Hepatitis C virus (HCV) also is carcinogenic and is associated with chronic hepatitis, cirrhosis, and liver cancer.

> A herpes virus (HHV-6) has recently been discovered to exist in Reed-Sternburg cells, which appear only in Hodgkin's disease, thus creating a causal association of the virus with the cancer. EBV also has been found in Reed-Sternburg cells. The DNA of HHV-6 has been implicated in adult T-cell lymphoblastic leukemia.

> HHV-8 has been shown to be the causative agent of Kaposi's sarcoma.

Sexual and Reproductive Behavior

Don't panic. Sex doesn't cause cancer. But certain sexual and reproductive behaviors and patterns tend to influence the risk of developing the disease. For example, circumcision greatly reduces a man's chance of penile cancer. In addition, their female sex partners have a lower risk of cervical cancer than do the partners of uncircumcised men. Sexual promiscuity, especially among women, increases exposure to the human papilloma virus, which is sexually transmitted and is closely associated with cervical cancer. And women who delay childbirth until later in life or who do not bear children at all are at increased risk of breast and ovarian cancer.

Electromagnetic Field Exposure

Electromagnetic fields (EMFs) are a combination of electric fields and magnetic fields that radiate from electric cables, power lines, and some electrical appliances and fixtures. Much has been written in the popular press recently about the links between EMF exposure and cancer. However, despite much observational data, there is no conclusive evidence that ordinary exposure to electromagnetic radiation at low frequencies, such as x-rays and ultraviolet radiation, causes cancer—or even has an association with the disease.

In terms of residential EMF, particular concern has centered around household appliances with which there is close personal contact: electric blankets, razors, hair dryers, and the like. But so far, no one has found any evidence that these appliances are risky, even with prolonged use.

In terms of occupational EMF, concern has centered around leukemia and brain cancer. But in all occupational studies conducted to date, none has shown a statistically significant risk increase except for a rise of 23 percent in brain cancer risk among welders. Even then, the risk of brain cancer for welders is negligible.

If EMF were to have a harmful effect, it would arise through stimulation of secondary electric currents in cell membranes and tissue fluids. EMF may amplify or otherwise affect normal electric currents in cells and tissues.

All observational data amassed has been epidemiological, not biological, because it would not be ethical to deliberately try to give people cancer by exposing them to high levels of EMF. Even so, none of the studies has provided persuasive results and all have been hampered by the fact that scientists cannot agree about what level of EMF might possibly be harmful. In addition, as a result of all studies conducted so far, scientific findings have concluded that a relationship between cancer (especially leukemia and brain cancer) is weak, inconsistent, and inconclusive.

Carcinogens in the Workplace

Much also has been written about the links between exposure to carcinogens in the workplace and cancer. However, here many of the associations are real, and there are definite cause-and-effect relationships between certain carcinogens (mostly chemicals) and cancer.

Although occupationally related cancers make up only a small percentage of all cancers—about 2 to 8 percent—in certain occupations in which workers are exposed to certain carcinogens, the risk is much higher. For more than two decades now, occupational environmentalists have been concerned about carcinogenicity for several reasons. First, if a chemical or other agent is carcinogenic, large numbers of people may be exposed to high concentrations of the agent. Second, the very nature of the workplace creates an ideal situation for studying cause-and-effect relationships between environmental exposure and cancer. Third, and probably most important, occupational cancers are, for the most part, entirely preventable by engineering for safety, establishing appropriate personnel practices, and enforcing strict protective legislation.

Of the more than 6 million identified chemicals, more than 50,000 are regularly used in commerce, and of those, fewer than 1,000 have been studied for their potential as carcinogens. About 120 are either known to be carcinogenic to humans or probably carcinogenic. Another 200 are possibly carcinogenic. Table 1-1 contains a partial list of the most common carcinogenic chemicals, the types of cancer they cause, and the usual ways they are used in commerce.

Table 1-1

Known and Suspected Chemical Carcinogens

Agent	Cancer	Commercial Use
Arsenic	Lung Skin	Metal smelting Electrical devices Semiconductors Medications Herbicides
Asbestos	Lung GI tract	Textiles Construction Friction materials Roofing materials Floor tiles
Benzene	Leukemia Hodgkin's Disease	Light oil Printing/lithography Paint Rubber Dry cleaning Detergents
Beryllium	Lung	Missile fuel Metal alloys
Cadmium	Prostate	Yellow pigments Solders/batteries
Chloromethyl methyl ether	Lung	Resins Industrial polymers Water repellents
Chromium compounds	Lung	Metal alloys Paints/pigments Preservatives
Diethylstilbesterol	Testis Vagina	Veterinary drugs Livestock feed
Ethylene oxide	Leukemia	Fruit ripening agent Rocket propellant Textile fumigation Hospital sterilant
Mustard gas	Lung	Poison war gas
Nickel compounds	Nose Lung	Nickel plating Ferrous alloys Ceramics Batteries
Vinyl chloride	Liver Angiosarcoma	Refrigerant Vinyl polymers Plastics adhesive

Metastasis

Metastasis means *spread*. Almost all cancers develop in one site. While they stay there, they are called cancer in situ. But eventually, they metastasize from there. The process consists of individual or small clumps of cells breaking off from the original tumor and traveling to other parts of the body. This happens in three major ways.

Direct extension is the way in which the tumor itself invades tissues and organs immediately adjacent to it—the way a can of spilled paint seeps into and around everything it touches until it is mopped up. *Hematogenous spread* is metastasis via the bloodstream, in which a tumor's own blood supply carries malignant cells to other parts of the body via the general circulation. A tumor also can metastasize via the *lymphatic system*, which is a system adjacent to the circulatory system designed to rid the body of waste products such as infections and toxic materials.

By and large, the older a cancer is, the more likely it is to have metastasized, which is why early diagnosis is so important to treatment success.

Cancer Growth Rate

The progress of cancer is measured not only by how far it has metastasized but also by how fast it is growing. This is done by means of a *biopsy*, a procedure in which a small piece of the tumor is surgically removed and examined under a microscope. The appearance and behavior of the tumor cells provide information about their type and rate of growth. It is also one way to determine the prognosis of the disease.

A number of characteristics identify cancer cells and help form a diagnosis and prognosis, as well as determine the type and course of treatment:

> ➤ *Well-differentiated* tumors look much like the normal tissue from which they arose. For example, cancerous tumor cells from the colon (large intestine) that are well-differentiated still look like colonic cells. A pathologist looking at these cells would know where they came from without being told.
> ➤ *Undifferentiated* tumors do not look like the normal tissue they came from. They are primitive, or immature, and a

pathologist probably would not be able to identify the tissue from which they arose. These tumors tend to be more aggressive, grow faster, and spread earlier than well-differentiated tumors.

➤ A *high-grade* tumor is immature, poorly differentiated, fast-growing, and aggressive.

➤ A *low-grade* tumor is usually mature, slow growing, well-differentiated, and less aggressive.

Staging

Staging is a way to determine how far the cancer has already progressed at the time of diagnosis, and it is generally the most important factor in determining treatment. The purposes of staging include identifying the extent of the disease: size, growth, and spread; estimating prognosis; and using a universal set of criteria against which all physicians can compare treatments.

Staging System

In recent years, a variety of staging systems has given way to one known as TNM (*T* stands for the size of the tumor, *N* for the degree of spread to lymph nodes, and *M* for the presence of metastasis). In addition, a number is added to each of the letters to indicate the stage of the tumor. For example, T0 means the tumor was completely removed by biopsy; T1 through T4 indicates the size of the tumor from smallest to largest; N0 means that nearby lymph nodes do not contain tumor cells; N1 through N4 indicates the degree of lymph node involvement, from least to most serious; M0 means that no metastasis has been found (not necessarily that it doesn't exist); and M1 indicates metastasis.

Diagnosis

Although the symptoms of cancer vary with the body part affected and the type of the disease, there are some general symptoms that are or may be indicative of cancer. These symptoms should not be ignored for two major reasons. First, if the problem is indeed cancer, it will only get worse. Second, the earlier a cancer is diagnosed, the easier it is to treat, and the more successful treatment will be. Following are some typical symptoms:

> ➤ *Unintended weight loss* may be an early symptom of cancer. It can be a symptom of many other problems or ailments as well, but it is not a normal occurrence.
> ➤ A *fever* is present in a majority of cancer patients, especially when the cancer arises from the lymphatic system or liver. Whenever the immune system is challenged (as when there is infection), the body temperature rises. Anyone with a fever who does not also have a cold or the flu should check with a physician.
> ➤ *Unexplained fatigue* that lingers longer than a person's lifestyle or recent life experiences warrants is possibly a symptom of cancer.
> ➤ Many cancers don't cause *pain* until they are well advanced, but some become painful in their earliest stages. This is true of sarcomas, and all cancers that begin in small places (such as eyes, brain, bladder, and chest) cause pain because they press on nearby nerves.
> ➤ Skin cancers are visually apparent in their very earliest stages and should not be ignored. Any *unexplained darkening of the skin* (hyperpigmentation), *new moles and other growths*, and *changes in existing moles or freckles* should be looked at right away by a dermatologist.

The earlier that cancer is diagnosed, the better the chances of remission and cure. The problem here is that most cancers do not produce symptoms until they are fairly far advanced. Still, various screening tests such as mammography, occult blood in the stool, and tumor marker assays can now detect the presence of some cancers in the very earliest stage.

However, most people don't bother with—and some don't have access to or can't afford—regular screening tests, so cancer diagnosis is still done the "old-fashioned" way: by noting signs and symptoms and performing tests to rule out other diseases and confirm the presence of a malignancy. Following are some of the tests and examinations done to detect the presence of cancer:

➤ Physical examination, in which symptoms are investigated by palpating, listening to, and looking at various body parts

➤ Blood tests

➤ Tumor marker assays, in which specific antigens (proteins) can be detected—for instance, prostate specific antigen (PSA), which can reveal the presence of prostate cancer

➤ Examination of body fluids (urine, spinal fluid, lymph, etc.) and stool to detect cancer cells

➤ Conventional radiography (x-ray) and digital radiography, which converts x-ray images into electronic data that can be viewed on a monitor and stored in a computer

➤ X-rays such as bone scans and barium contrast pictures

➤ Imaging techniques such as *computerized tomography (CT scan)* and *magnetic resonance imaging (MRI)*, which uses a confluence of electromagnets and radio waves to produce a computerized picture of internal organs and structures that pinpoint the location of tumors

➤ Radioisotope scans, which also show tumor location

➤ *Angiography*, in which dye is injected into blood vessels to determine their size, shape, and patency

➤ *Ultrasonography*, which creates a picture on a monitor from a reflection of sound waves passed through the body and detects structural or functional abnormalities

➤ Various scoping devices in which a flexible tube with a *fiberoptic* light attached is inserted into a body orifice to visualize tubelike structures (trachea, lungs, rectum, colon, etc.)

➤ *Cytological* studies, which is an examination of cellular material to identify cancer cells as defined previously

➤ Bone marrow analysis to determine the nature of abnormal blood-producing cells

➤ Biopsy, in which a small piece of the tumor is surgically removed and examined under a microscope to perform cytological studies to identify tumor cells

Chapter Two

Chemotherapy

How and Why Drugs and Drug Combinations Kill Cancer Cells

*E*ven if a course or courses of chemotherapy does not cure your cancer (five years of complete remission is generally used as a benchmark for a cure), it can provide many months or years of productive, normal life. Moreover, it can improve the quality of that life by significantly relieving pain and other symptoms. In fact, many types of cancer can be cured or well treated in so many instances that they are now thought of as chronic rather than acute (and usually terminal) illnesses. Although the decision to undergo chemotherapy is yours—and yours alone—if your physician suggests it, think positively about the opportunity you are being offered. Chemotherapy is certainly not an enjoyable experience, but in the long run you will be far better off.

Once a cell has mutated into a cancerous form, the set of instructions contained in its DNA is irrevocably altered, and it will never again behave like a normal cell. The *only* course of action is to kill it.

In general, chemotherapy works by interfering with cells' DNA, especially the reproductive function. Drugs are either cycle specific (they kill cells only during a specific phase of reproduction), or they are cycle nonspecific (they can kill cells regardless of the reproductive cycle). One is not necessarily better or more effective than the other.

For *cytotoxic* (cell killing) chemotherapy to be effective, it must have the capacity to do several things. A drug must reach the cells it is designed to kill, and a sufficiently high dose must enter the cancer cells and remain there for a long enough time to kill them. In addition, the cancer cells themselves must be sufficiently sensitive to the effects of the drug and must remain so until they become resistant to the drug (see the following sections for more about drug resistance). This is a little like the weeds in a garden. Some die easily when sprayed with weed killer, and some eventually get used to and adapt to the poison and continue to thrive.

Making the Chemotherapy Decision

The decision to embark on a course of chemotherapy is yours alone, of course, but you owe it to yourself to make that decision as sensibly as possible. Chemotherapy is not the be-all and end-all of your newly diagnosed cancer, or that of someone close to you, but it can be a life-changing adventure—and a life-saving one.

Chemotherapy is not a day at the beach. Nor is it just a minor inconvenience. It's serious stuff, and although you certainly won't experience all the side effects discussed in Chapter 7, you will have some of them. There will be days when you'll wonder what all the fuss is about, and other days when you will feel wretched. There may even be times when you will feel tempted to say, "Enough! I can't do this anymore." But don't give up. Keep reminding yourself that chemotherapy doesn't last forever, and that when it's over you will most likely be far better off than you were.

When you first receive your diagnosis, and for several days thereafter, you will feel so overwhelmed with the fact of having cancer that you may not feel capable of making a decision. But as soon as the shock wears off, and when you begin to discuss your disease and your feelings about it with people you feel close to, you will need to find out what you'll be getting into—what chemotherapy entails—so you'll have the information you need to make a sensible, informed decision.

Ask your oncologist right away about the following:

1. The pros and cons of the specific treatment he or she is suggesting
2. The statistical chance of the treatment's success (numbers don't mean everything, but they *are* a good indication of probable success)
3. The alternatives to the recommended treatment

4. The logistical details—where the treatment is given, how often you'll have to receive treatment, how long it will last, how it's administered, and how much it will cost

Then, as you think about what to do, as well as during the course of the treatment, other questions will occur to you. Write them down so you don't forget, and *do* ask your physician or the office staff (who often know more about the ancillary details than the doctor does) whatever you want to know—and make certain you understand the answer.

The decision about which drug or drugs to use is your physician's, not yours. But as a cancer patient you should be aware of the factors that go into making that decision: the stage of the disease at diagnosis; predictions of the direction in which the tumor might spread; and the risk-to-benefit ratio—that is, how much good the drug will do as compared with the number and severity of side effects and what you are willing and able to tolerate.

A number of factors go into making the decision about how to treat cancer. The *stage*—that is, the progress of the cancer at the time of diagnosis—is probably the most critical factor. The *type* of cancer also affects the decision. Certain types of cancer have an affinity for certain other tissues (for example, prostate cancer likes bone tissue, as does breast cancer; and ovarian cancer often spreads to the brain), but wherever it goes, the cells remain the same type. In other words, metastasized prostate cancer always looks like prostate cancer even when it has moved to bone tissue. Your physicians need to know the type of cells they are dealing with when choosing chemotherapeutic drugs.

The *biology of the disease*—that is, the cell types and their expected behavior—is also part of the decision. So are personal factors such as *age, general health, other accompanying medical conditions*, and *family history of cancer*.

Tumor Boards

A *tumor board* is a group of oncologists and other physicians who meet regularly in all cancer hospitals, as well as at other major medical centers, to discuss patients' progress and to determine the advantages and disadvantages of various courses of treatment. Your physician may present your case (anonymously, of course) if he or she has questions or comments, if your case is unusual in any way, or if treatment has been exceptional. A pathologist will bring copies of your biopsy report, your x-rays will be highlighted in light boxes, and a nuclear medicine specialist will talk about your various scans.

The advantage of a tumor board is that your physician has an opportunity to benefit from the thinking of other cancer specialists, and the pros and cons of a variety of types of chemotherapeutic agents are discussed. You may or may not be told that your case has been presented. However, whatever the board thinks is to your best advantage, the decision to participate in any treatment always remains yours.

Classes of Drugs

Chemotherapeutic drugs and other agents (which are called *biologicals* and will be described in Chapter 4) are designed to interfere with the cycle of abnormal cancer cell growth and change. That is the major and only purpose, but different classes of drugs accomplish the goal in different ways.

Antimetabolites

Antimetabolites attack cells as they are dividing (so they are *cycle specific*), which is when they are especially vulnerable. Their main mechanism of action is interference with the synthesis of DNA and RNA (ribonucleic acid), and they also mimic the normal chemical structure of *metabolites* (the changed end products of nutrients that are necessary for normal cell metabolism). They are most effective against rapidly growing cells, and they prohibit cell replication by deceiving cells into incorporating them along certain metabolic pathways that are essential for synthesis of RNA or DNA so that a false genetic message is transmitted. In essence, antimetabolite drugs "trick" cells into ingesting them—and then they turn around and kill the cells.

Some antimetabolites inhibit enzymes that are necessary for synthesis of essential cell chemicals. In other words, they block cancer cells' ability to carry out life processes—so they die. Because antimetabolites have such a small window of opportunity to kill cells, the longer these drugs are given, the more cells they will be able to kill.

Antimetabolites, because they act on rapidly dividing cells, cause the most toxicity in normal cells that also divide rapidly: those of the oral mucosa, bone marrow stem cells, and cells of the gastrointestinal tract.

Some of the more commonly used antimetabolites include cytabarine, fluorouracil, gemcitabine, mercaptopurine, and methotrexate.

Alkylating Agents

Alkylating agents (also called DNA cross-linking agents) attack all cells in a tumor regardless of whether they are resting or dividing, although they cause the greatest damage to cells when they are active. They bind with the cells' DNA in various ways to prevent reproduction. In addition, they cause breaks in DNA strands, which are then unable to separate, which in turn prevents replication of cellular genetic material. Alkylating agents are *cycle nonspecific*; that is, they exert their effect on all parts of the cell cycle (the life phases of all cells are growth, division, and rest), but they are most effective against rapidly dividing cells.

Alkylating agents are used to reduce the size of tumors (a process called *debulking*), which causes resting cells to begin active division. As a result, those cells are vulnerable to cycle-specific drugs, with which alkylating agents are often used in combination. Alkylating agents are especially active against lymphomas, Hodgkin's disease, breast cancer, and multiple myeloma.

The downside of alkylating agents is that when they are given at high doses, there is an increased risk of developing secondary malignancies (which are other primary tumors), such as bladder cancer and leukemia. In addition, some alkylating agents negatively affect bone marrow stem cells, causing deficiency in certain white cells, called myelosuppression (see Chapter 7 for a thorough discussion of drug toxicities). They also can cause changes in testicular and ovarian function, which negatively affects sperm and egg production and which can take several years to return to normal.

Some of the more commonly used alkylating agents include busulfan, carboplatin, cisplatin, cyclophosphamide, leukeran, mustargen, procarbazine, and thiotepa.

Anti-tumor Antibiotics

Anti-tumor antibiotics, agents isolated from living microorganisms, insert themselves into cell DNA to break up the chromosomes or to inhibit synthesis of RNA that cells require for continued growth. This process is similar to, but much more aggressive than, the process you are used to with various antibiotics used to treat bacterial infections.

Different antibiotics produce cytotoxic effects (killing cells) in different ways. For example, anthracyclines such as daunomycin and doxorubicin cause DNA strands to break, some prevent DNA synthesis, and others cause cell membrane function to change. Mitomycin also is an alkylator (see the previous section), and mithramycin inhibits DNA-directed RNA synthesis. Most anti-tumor antibiotics are cell cycle nonspecific.

Major side effects are myelosuppression; skin and gastrointestinal problems; cardiac problems; and liver, kidney, and blood clotting dysfunction.

Plant Alkaloids and Other Natural Products

Plant (vinca) alkaloids, also called *mitotic inhibitors* (such as vincristine, vinblastine, teniposide, etoposide, paclitaxel, and docetaxel), disturb chromosome formation and thus interrupt or prevent cell duplication. They also crystallize certain proteins, which arrests cell division and thus kills the cell. Plant alkaloids are cycle-specific drugs. Major side effects include myelosuppression and neurological problems.

Topoisomerase inhibitors (such as camptothecin, topotecan, and irinotecan) are enzymes that break up and reconfigure strands of DNA in order to interfere with cell replication.

Enzymes such as L-aspariginase inhibit protein synthesis by depriving tumor cells of the amino acid asparagine. Normal cells can produce their own asparagine, but malignant cells cannot and are therefore adversely affected by L-asparaginase.

Hormones and Other Endocrine Drugs

Hormones inhibit the growth of some cancers, although no one yet knows exactly how. One theory is that some tumors depend on existing in a certain hormonal environment, and when that environment is changed, tumor growth is altered or arrested. However, using hormones or hormone antagonists to treat cancer depends on the presence of hormone receptors in the tumor itself. Breast, thyroid, prostate, and uterine cancers are particularly sensitive to hormonal manipulation.

Commonly used hormones include estrogens, anti-estrogens such as tamoxifen, androgens, and corticosteroids such as prednisone. They are given alone or in combination with other drugs. In rare instances, the "offending" endocrine gland (from which hormones are secreted) is removed, and cytotoxic drugs are administered before or after surgery—or both.

The side effects of hormonal therapy result from using higher doses than the body requires for normal function. They include, depending on the hormone, changes in secondary sex characteristics, changes in libido, fluid retention, hypertension (high blood pressure), hyperglycemia (too much glucose in the bloodstream), ulcers, osteoporosis, increased appetite, susceptibility to infection, and others.

Miscellaneous Agents

Miscellaneous agents are those whose mechanism of action does not fall into one of the other classes of anticancer drugs (also called *antineoplastic* drugs). They include L-asparaginase, mitotane, mitoxantrone, procarbazine, and paclitaxel.

You can find a complete list of all cancer drugs in Appendix A. They are arranged by the classifications listed here and are cross-referenced by the type of cancer for which they are usually given.

Combination Chemotherapy

Most cancer chemotherapy consists of two or more drugs given in *combination*, either at the same time or sequentially. For instance, drugs that attack tumor cells at all stages of their life cycle may be given first to shrink the tumor, which makes the remaining cells divide. When they do, the second, cycle-specific drug will attack cells as they too divide. Other sequences of other drugs maximize this effect. In general, combination chemotherapy is much more effective than the use of a single agent; it produces less overall toxicity (serious side effects); and, except in rare instances, it has replaced single-agent therapy, which rarely led to complete responses. By targeting different biochemical processes, it has become possible to achieve complete, long-lasting remission and even to cure some types of advanced cancer.

In the 1960s, when cancer research moved into high gear and many new drugs were in the research pipeline, the disadvantages of single-agent chemotherapy became apparent. First, it was difficult to achieve long-term remission. Second, tumor cells quickly became resistant to further chemotherapy; this was the most common reason for treatment failure. Third, single agents produced severe or lethal toxicity when given in high enough doses to kill cancer cells.

One of the earliest successes of combination chemotherapy is the Cooper regimen for advanced breast cancer. It consists of cyclophosphamide, methotrexate, 5-FU, vincristine, and predinsone. Shortly thereafter, MOPP therapy (mechlorethamine, vincristine [also known as oncovin], procarbazine, and prednisone) was developed for Hodgkin's disease. They are both still in wide use today, as are dozens of other combinations. New combinations are being developed all the time.

Combination chemotherapy uses both the additive and *synergistic* effects of two or more drugs. *Additive* simply means that a patient receives the benefits of both drugs at once—a kind of "two for the price of one" deal. *Synergistic* means that the total effect of two or more drugs adds up to more than the sum of the total—"three for the price of two." That is, each drug, when combined with another, provides greater therapeutic effect than it would on its own.

In general, the advantages of combination chemotherapy are that it allows for maximum cell kill without *dose-limiting toxicity* (so many and such serious side effects that the dose has to be reduced); it creates a broader range of coverage for resistant tumor cells; it prevents or slows the development of resistant cells; and it uses intermittent treatment schedules, which permits the recovery of normal tissues between treatment cycles.

In designing drug combinations, three approaches can be used. The *biochemical approach* means that by using drugs that damage cancer cells in different ways, one can attack or inhibit different biochemical processes that the cells require to live and/or reproduce. The goal of this approach is to decrease production of the products that the tumor needs for growth and development.

The *cytokinetic approach* means that drugs produce changes in cells that make them more vulnerable to cycle-specific agents. For example, debulking a tumor with chemotherapy increases the percentage of the actively dividing cells that remain, which then are more easily killed by cycle-specific drugs.

The *empirical approach* means that the different mechanisms of action of the drugs in the combination complement one another to kill the maximum number of cells. An advantage of this approach is that the toxicities of individual drugs usually differ, which means that the drugs can be administered at nearly full tolerated doses without severe side effects. Combination chemotherapy reduces the chance of cells becoming resistant to a particular drug.

How does an oncologist decide which combination to use for which cancer—in which patient? Experience and the results of randomized clinical trials provide the best answers, which is one of the most compelling reasons to participate in a clinical trial (see Chapter 6). Some of the combinations offer no real survival advantage, especially in patients who have "failed" other drug regimens, but many provide excellent palliation. Some combinations provide "salvage" therapy for patients who have failed other regimens but who do not want to give up the effort to treat the disease, and others are good *second-line treatment* for patients who, for a variety of reasons, cannot take the preferred treatment.

Drug Resistance

Just as antibiotics or pain medications sometimes fail to work, so too with chemotherapy. There are many reasons why this happens. If the cancer is far advanced and/or growing extremely rapidly, cytotoxic drugs are less likely to be effective. In addition, the greater the number of actively reproducing cells a tumor has, the greater the chance that they will be only minimally affected by chemotherapy. If insufficient amounts of the drug reach the tumor, as may happen if there is a poor blood supply, efficacy will be diminished.

But by far the biggest reason for the failure of chemotherapy is drug *resistance*, either because some cancer cells are intrinsically resistant (and thus are never affected by a particular chemotherapeutic agent), or because, over a period of time, they adapt themselves to the presence of a drug and are no longer sensitive to it. The phenomenon of resistance is not fully understood, but there are a number of theories about why it happens.

One theory is that transport of the drug into cancer cells via the bloodstream becomes defective, so that more of the drug is excreted (eliminated from the body, most often in the urine and feces) before it is used by the cells. Cellular concentration is thus diminished. In addition, the metabolism of the drug may be defective; the drug may become inactive; the cancer cells' DNA may "learn" how to repair the damage caused by the drug; or the drug target inside the cells may become altered so that the drug can no longer recognize it.

There are, however, tests that can determine degrees of resistance so the problem can be caught early and, to a great extent, averted.

High-dose Chemotherapy

High-dose chemotherapy (also called *dose-intensive chemotherapy*) is designed to destroy cancer cells more effectively than standard doses of drugs. The theory is that increasing dose intensity will provide a higher cumulative dose in a shorter period of time and thus result in increased tumor-cell kill. However, while a drug attacks tumor cells, it also destroys bone marrow. Therefore, bone marrow transplantation is often used in conjunction with high-dose chemotherapy (see Chapter 5).

The treatment regimen called high-dose chemotherapy is fairly new. It consists of giving greatly increased doses of cell cycle-dependent drugs (alkylating agents are usually best) in an effort to cure malignancies that have not been curable with standard doses. In addition, plant alkaloids (etoposide, teniposide, and paclitaxel, for example) are being used in combination with alkylating agents and have produced some excellent results. Toxic side effects may or may not also increase.

Sometimes *stem cells* (immature blood-forming cells) are removed before high-dose chemotherapy is given. The stem cells are preserved and then, in an attempt to re-establish normal blood production, are given back to the patient after the course of chemotherapy is over. See Chapter 5 for more detail.

The therapy is given for one or more cycles, and because it sometimes causes severe side effects (many of which can be minimized with medications given before or during the therapy), you may need to be hospitalized or find a place to stay that is close to the hospital so you can get there without delay. The most common side effects are nausea and vomiting, diarrhea, mouth sores, skin rash, and hair loss.

Treatment Goals

Talking about treatment goals in cancer chemotherapy may at first seem like a "no-brainer." The goal is to cure the disease. Right? Yes, but it's not that simple. Although many cancers are indeed curable, many are not. However, even though a cancer may not be definitively cured does not mean that embarking on a course of chemotherapy is futile. In the vast majority of cases, chemotherapy is positive and worthwhile.

Chemotherapy is used to treat both early—almost invisible— tumors as well as larger ones, although it is usually most effective on rapidly growing cancers, such as lymphomas and leukemias, in which cells divide and reproduce quickly. It is least effective on the slowest-growing tumors, such as prostate cancer.

In addition to curing the patient, there are a number of other treatment goals. Tumor growth can be controlled when a cure isn't possible, which provides additional survival time. Symptoms such as pain can be relieved. Tumors can be significantly shrunk prior to surgery or radiation therapy, which makes those treatments more effective. Microscopic metastases can be destroyed after tumors are surgically removed, which is known as *adjuvant therapy*. Metastasis or recurrence of the disease often can be prevented.

Once you begin treatment, you'll hear the phrase *adjuvant chemotherapy* a good deal. It sounds more complex than it is. *Adjuvant* simply means a treatment, in this case chemotherapy, that is used in addition to and following primary treatment to cure the cancer, reduce the number of stray metastatic cells, or palliate symptoms. Adjuvant chemotherapy is most commonly used after surgery, but it is also used after first-line chemotherapy itself, most often if the patient didn't respond adequately to the first attempt.

Giving adjuvant therapy as a kind of "mop-up" measure after surgery seems so obviously a good idea that it is surprising that only in the past decade or so has it been tested and proven efficacious by clinical trials (first in breast cancer) to cure disease or result in long-term remission.

What Happens as a Result of Chemotherapy

Four major things happen as a result of chemotherapy. *Complete remission*, also called *complete response*, means that the tumor disappears entirely—either permanently or for a very long time. *Partial remission*, or *partial response*, means that the tumor shrinks significantly but does not disappear. *Stabilization* means that the tumor neither shrinks nor grows. *Progression* means that the tumor continues to grow despite chemotherapy.

Measuring the Response to Chemotherapy

The ways to determine if a tumor is responding to chemotherapy are similar to the ways in which the cancer was diagnosed in the first place:

> ➤ Direct measurement of the tumor or lymph nodes either by palpation or x-ray
> ➤ CT scans and MRIs used to measure deep internal tumors that cannot be palpated or visualized by ordinary x-ray
> ➤ Tumor marker tests and other blood assays
> ➤ Assessment of Karnofsky Performance Status, a measurement of one's ability to function normally

Selecting Drugs

The way your physician chooses your drugs depends on a variety of factors. He or she looks at the statistical probability that the course of treatment will work for you. There is no foolproof way to predict the future, of course, but other peoples' past experience with the same type of cancer is a strong indication of success. The stage of your tumor, your age, your general physical health, and other accompanying medical problems affect the choice of drugs. The sensitivity of various tumors to various drugs, which is determined by a laboratory test of *your* tumor cells on a particular drug or combination, is established. This is called a *clonigenic assay*. The possibility of using other types of treatment along with or instead of chemotherapy is also assessed for cancers that respond well to a number of different treatments, such as breast cancer.

Dosage

In general, the larger the dose of a chemotherapeutic agent, the more malignant cells it will kill—and the more toxic effects it will produce. Therefore, a balance must be established between effective chemotherapy and the ability to tolerate side effects. Several considerations are involved in determining dosage. First, avoiding all, or even most, toxic effects is not a desirable goal because too low a dose will not have the desired anticancer effect and will reduce the possibility of cure or remission. Second, the *maximum safe dose* for cure is the most effective dose. *Safety* and *efficacy* are the key words here. Third, occasionally a drug is too toxic to healthy cells even as it produces the desired effect on cancer cells. In this event, the drug must be discontinued and you will be switched to another. However, deciding how much toxicity is "too toxic" is not a cut-and-dried decision, nor is it an easy one to make.

Administration

Chemotherapy is almost always administered in a series of *cycles*: a period of several days or weeks in which you receive the drug, followed by a period of rest. In rare instances, people receive chemotherapy as a inpatient, but most often it is done on an outpatient basis, either at the hospital or in your doctor's office. Drugs are administered in a variety of ways, and the route of administration depends largely on the goal of the chemotherapy and the form of the drug in which it is manufactured.

There are two general approaches to drug delivery: *systemic* and *regional*. *Systemic administration*, which is the most common form of cancer chemotherapy, includes *oral*; *subcutaneous* (injected just under the skin); *intramuscular* (injected deep into a large muscle like the upper thigh or buttocks); and *intravenous* (into a vein). The intravenous route of systemic administration is the most usual for cancer chemotherapy.

Regional approaches include *intraperitoneal* (into the abdomen); *intravesical* (into the urinary bladder); *intrathecal* (into the spinal fluid); *intra-arterial* (into an artery); *intrapleural* (into the covering of the lungs); and *topical* (rubbed onto the skin). The most commonly administered routes are described in detail as follows:

➤ *Oral treatment*, by mouth in pill or capsule form, is the eas-
iest and most palatable way to administer chemotherapy, but
drug absorption can be inconsistent depending on the condition of the stomach and small intestine as well as other factors. Moreover, some patients have trouble sticking to a
dosing schedule, which can seriously affect the drug's efficacy and safety.

➤ *Intravenous delivery*, in which the drug is infused via a needle
inserted into a vein, is the way chemotherapeutic drugs are
usually given. Sometimes, when veins are too small or too
often used, a tiny plastic tube (called a *catheter*) is attached to
the needle and threaded through to a larger vein. The infusion
lasts anywhere from 15 minutes to 8 hours, with an average
of 90 minutes. A series of infusions, given once a week or
several times a week, is called a *cycle*. Intravenous infusion
provides consistency of dosing, but side effects, such as scle-
rosing (hardening) of veins, infection, and phlebitis (inflammation of veins) are almost inevitable over time.

➤ *Peripheral venous access*—in which a long catheter called a
PICC line (peripherally inserted central catheter) is inserted
into the basilic or cephalic vein in the arm and threaded up to
the superior vena cava (a major vein) near the heart—
bypasses some of the most serious problems of intravenous
delivery. The catheter, with an access port on the outside of
the skin, is left in place for the duration of the chemotherapy.
Insertion of the PICC line is done in the x-ray department
because ultrasound is used to help guide the catheter through
the veins. The procedure is painless, except for the initial stick
of the needle, and some people find it fascinating to watch the
catheter snake through their circulatory system. But you
don't have to look if you don't want to.

➤ A *central venous catheter* is similar to a PICC, but it is inserted
into the circulatory system through the chest wall through
subcutaneous tissue and into a large blood vessel such as the
superior vena cava. This procedure is more complex than
PICC insertion and is done in the operating room under general or local anesthesia. Central venous catheters are accompanied by a few complications: they can become occluded or

cause an infection; they can cause a clot or an air embolism; and they can break or perforate the vein.

➤ An *infusion port* is a device placed under the skin at one of a variety of sites; it serves as a reservoir for the drug. A catheter leads from the port into a large vein. The drug to be administered is injected into the port from which it flows outward into the circulation. An infusion port has to be inserted—and removed—surgically, but after it is in place, you hardly know it's there, and because the risk of infection is very low, it can stay in place for many months—even years. It will not restrict your activities and requires minimal patient maintenance. The biggest disadvantage is that a needle puncture (just under the skin, not into the vein) is required for each dose of medication. Also, the catheter can become clogged so the drug backs up into the port, or it can leak, which can damage the vein.

➤ An *ambulatory pump* delivers the chemotherapy while you go about your regular activities. The pump holds the drug or drugs and is attached to a catheter that goes into your body via a needle and catheter apparatus.

➤ *Central nervous system delivery* is done via a lumbar puncture (called *intrathecal administration*), which is not as bad as it sounds, but it's not a picnic, either. A catheter is threaded through the needle and chemotherapy is administered that way. Another method of central nervous system delivery is the Ommaya reservoir, a dome-shaped device placed under the scalp and connected to a hollow section in the brain that contains cerebrospinal fluid. It is inserted in the operating room under local anesthesia. Once the pump is in place and the sutures have healed, it is left there permanently, and there's nothing special the patient has to do about it. There are a number of possible complications (infection, malfunction, catheter displacement, and the spread of tumor cells by the placement of the catheter), but they are not common.

➤ *Intraperitoneal administration* means that drugs are delivered directly into the abdomen. This route is used most often when there is abdominal metastasis, usually from the colon or ovary. The major advantage is that high concentrations of some drugs can be administered, but this also carries a disadvantage: high drug concentrations can result in greater toxicity.

➤ *The intra-arterial method* delivers drugs to a specific organ or part of the body via a major artery supplying the organ or part. Intra-arterial infusion has been used for head and neck cancer, but the liver is the primary site. Chemotherapy can be delivered via an externally placed catheter, an implanted port, or an implanted pump. Intra-arterial perfusion catheters are inserted in the hospital under local anesthesia. This method of chemotherapy administration is not used often because the procedure is so complex and the complication rate so high.

Duration of Treatment

Treatment lasts until you have responded to the fullest extent possible, until the drugs become too toxic, or until your physician thinks you will do better on a different drug or combination. This is not meant to sound simplistic, but it does illustrate how individual and ever-changing cancer chemotherapy can be. There are indeed standard courses of treatment for most drugs, but individual human beings do not always conform to standards, and a good oncologist will start out with the most aggressive standard treatment available and then will carefully monitor your progress and make changes as necessary.

In general, however, length of treatment depends on the therapy program. Most programs last from about six months to a year. When remission has been achieved, treatment is continued for a bit longer in an attempt to kill undetectable cells. When chemotherapy is combined with radiotherapy, specific rules and formulas apply that may differ somewhat from chemotherapy alone.

Adjuvant chemotherapy may be given for six months to a year after surgery or after primary chemotherapy is stopped. This is designed to kill small nests of undetected cells.

Chapter Three

Blood Components

All Blood Cells Are Affected by the Cancer and the Drugs Used to Treat It

When you are diagnosed with cancer, one of the many things you will feel like is a pincushion. From the time the diagnosis is sought until after treatment is finished, physicians, nurses, and laboratory technicians will be after you for blood samples. Constantly holding out your arm for a needle stick gets very old, very fast, and it's one of the things that people hate most about having cancer. You know that all the blood testing is necessary, but that doesn't mean you have to like it, and you may not know why. All the tests are necessary.

The Function of Blood

Blood is the body's most important fluid, and it flows to every single cell in your body. It has a number of vital functions. The bloodstream picks up oxygen from the lungs and circulates it to the cells. Without oxygen, cells die. Cells also need glucose for energy, which the blood collects from the liver and other organs and delivers to them. Blood contains the cells that are the body's defense against infection. It also contains a wide variety of other chemicals and hormones needed to maintain physical function.

Components of Blood

Blood consists of cells and *plasma*. Plasma is a yellowish fluid in which the cells, enzymes, minerals, vitamins, hormones, and other chemicals float. A *complete blood count* (CBC) examines the cells, and a *blood chemistry* tests plasma. You will have both tests many, many times.

Bone Marrow

Bone marrow, the soft tissue at the core of some bones, is a blood cell manufacturing plant. In adults, cells are produced only in the flat bones of the pelvis, breastbone (sternum), and skull. In infants, cells are produced in all marrow.

The marrow makes immature blood cells, called *stem cells*, which develop into one of three types: red blood cells, white blood cells, or platelets. Marrow is in a continuous production mode; as old cells die off, it makes new ones, and it can step up production when there is a special need, such as in the event of an infection when white cells are required to attack bacteria, viruses, and other toxic material.

In a bone marrow biopsy, a needle is inserted into the hipbone (iliac crest), breastbone (sternum), or backbone (vertebra), and marrow tissue is aspirated in much the same way as blood is aspirated after a needle is inserted into a vein. Of course, in bone marrow biopsy, the needle has to be inserted more deeply, so the skin and tissue over the bone is anesthetized. The tissue is then spread on slides and sent to the laboratory for examination.

Effect of Chemotherapy on Bone Marrow

Since marrow consists of cells that are immature and divide quickly, and because cancer drugs attack rapidly dividing cells, bone marrow is strongly affected by chemotherapy. One of the reasons why chemotherapy is given in cycles is to allow the bone marrow time to recover, which it usually does in a week to 10 days.

Red Blood Cells

Red cells (*erythrocytes*), which give blood its color, consist almost entirely of *hemoglobin* (90 percent). Hemoglobin is a substance rich in iron to which oxygen adheres as it is carried to cells. Red blood cells (RBCs) are shaped like dinner plates (round and slightly convex); an abnormal shape or fragmented cells suggest the presence of disease such as iron or vitamin deficiency. Normal RBC count is 4.5–5 million.

RBCs comprise about half the blood's volume, and each cell lives for about 30 days. New RBCs are continuously manufactured to replace ones that die. Death and production of all blood cells is a normal process.

Reticulocytes are newly formed (young) red blood cells, which comprise about 1 percent of the total RBCs. When the body needs more red cells, as it does when anemia (a common side effect of some chemotherapy) is present, the bone marrow produces more reticulocytes. Therefore, the reticulocyte count is one measure of bone marrow function, an important piece of information during the course of chemotherapy.

Effect of Chemotherapy on Red Cells

Production of RBCs diminishes and results in a condition called *anemia*, and the most noticeable symptom is fatigue. Transfusions of whole blood or packed red cells are sometimes (but not often) necessary. A substance called erythropoietin can stimulate the production of red cells. (See Chapter 4 for a discussion of blood growth factors.)

White Blood Cells

White blood cells (*leukocytes*) are less numerous than RBCs (the ratio is about 1:660). Their primary purpose is to defend the body against infection—and to fight infection when it occurs, including production of antibodies. Five types of white cells are produced in the bone marrow, and separating white cells into their components is called a *differential blood count*. You'll hear doctors talk about it as "the diff." Normal WBC count is 4,500–10,500. Following are the five types:

> *Neutrophils* (also called *granulocytes*), the most common type of WBC, localize and neutralize bacteria and fungi. They also ingest foreign cells. Neutrophils are divided into band (immature) and segmented (mature) cells.
> *Eosinophils* respond to allergic reactions, kill some parasites, and destroy some cancer cells.

➤ *Basophils* release histamine (part of the allergic response), which increases blood supply and attracts other white cells to an infected area.

➤ *Lymphocytes* fight infection, as well as provide immunity to certain diseases. They react to foreign substances and form antibodies. T-lymphocytes (also called *T-cells*) help protect against viral infections and can detect and destroy some cancer cells. B-lymphocytes (*B-cells*) develop into cells that produce antibodies that attack foreign substances. Each B-cell is designed to produce one specific antibody to fight one specific foreign substance—a bacterium or virus, for example.

➤ *Monocytes* react more slowly than neutrophils and are thus the second line of defense against infection. They ingest damaged or dying cells and provide some immunologic protection.

Effect of Chemotherapy on White Cells

White cell production is extremely vulnerable to chemotherapy, partly because white cells normally live only three or four days, thus creating a serious risk of infection. White cell counts usually drop to their lowest point (called the *nadir*) about a week to 10 days after a cycle of chemotherapy and come back to normal about three weeks after treatment. Your count will be checked before you begin the next cycle.

If the production of white cells does not recover spontaneously, you may be given one or more of a number of types of a genetically engineered protein called *colony-stimulating factor* (see Chapter 4). This stimulates production of white cells.

Platelets

Platelets (*thrombocytes*) play a significant role in blood clot formation. They clump together at the site of an internal or external injury and make blood vessels constrict. They then engage in a series of chemical reactions and interact with other clotting factors in the plasma, as well as substances they themselves release. Normal platelet count is 200,000–350,000.

Effect of Chemotherapy on Platelets

Chemotherapy slows platelet production. The lowest number of circulating platelets occurs about two weeks following chemotherapy, but it almost always returns to normal spontaneously. The noticeable effect of a low platelet count is that you may bruise more readily, and your mucous membranes are more likely to bleed, such as when you brush your teeth and use dental floss.

Plasma

Plasma is the fluid in which red and white cells and platelets float. It also contains a number of other substances:

➤ *Electrolytes* are the chemicals that your body requires in order to function. They include sodium, potassium, chloride, and calcium.
➤ *Proteins* are large molecules, such as albumen and globulin, that control the flow of fluid from the circulatory system to the cells.
➤ Various *enzymes* are required by the heart and liver to function normally.
➤ *Clotting factors* work with platelets to stop bleeding.
➤ Substances such as nitrogen, urea, and creatinine are needed for proper kidney function.

Tumor Markers

A recent development in cancer research is the discovery of *tumor markers* (also called *biological markers*). These are substances (*antigens*) released by some cancers into the bloodstream. Their presence at abnormally high levels often (but not always) indicates development of a malignancy. They do not constitute foolproof diagnosis, but they are an important diagnostic tool.

Tumor marker tests are expensive and not very specific. Therefore, they are not especially valuable as screening devices, but they are being used in diagnosis and treatment of cancer, especially in determining if treatment has been successful. If the marker disappears from the bloodstream, the indication is that treatment has probably been successful.

One of the best-known tumor markers is prostate specific antigen (PSA), an elevated level of which may indicate the presence of prostate cancer. Others include the following:

➤ Carcinoembryonic antigen (CEA) is found in the blood of people with cancer of the colon, breast, pancreas, bladder, ovary, and cervix. However, high levels of CEA also are secreted by people who are heavy smokers and those who have cirrhosis of the liver or ulcerative colitis, so the presence of CEA does not necessarily indicate cancer, and false positives are very common.

➤ Alpha-fetoprotein (AFP), normally produced by fetal liver cells, is often found in people with cancer of the ovary or testis.

➤ Beta-human chorionic gonadotropin (B-HCG) is a hormone produced during pregnancy and secreted by women with cancer originating in the placenta and by men with testicular cancer.

➤ CA-125 is an antigen secreted in a variety of ovarian diseases, including cancer.

➤ CA-15-3 is found in people with breast cancer.

➤ CA-19-5 is found in people with pancreatic cancer.

Chapter Four

Biological Therapy

Using Genetic Engineering to Attack Cancer Where It Starts

Biological Therapy

Biological therapy means using genetic engineering (creating or manipulating genes in the laboratory) and other redirections of natural cells and substances to treat disease, in this case cancer. Many of the treatments now being studied in the laboratory and in patients stimulate the immune system with engineered purified proteins to activate the body's natural defenses to kill cancer cells. What this means for cancer therapy is that scientists are trying to unlock the secrets of the body's genetic code and immune system in order to attack cancer at its source: in the very cells where it arises.

Before we talk about *genetics* and biological therapy, you may need a review of what a *gene* is. It is the biologic unit of heredity, and there are thousands of genes on the *chromosomes* in the nucleus of each and every cell in the body. As you may remember from high school biology, there are 23 matched pairs of chromosomes, and each gene contains a blueprint for the manufacture of a particular protein, which in turn is responsible for one inherited trait. Genes that have minor abnormalities are called *oncogenes*, and they can cause developmental defects, some of which may lead to or cause cancer. We will discuss the physical and biochemical nature of genes in more detail throughout this chapter.

Biological therapy is designed to work in a number of different ways: by enhancing the immune system; by making cancer cells more sensitive to destruction by the immune system; by stimulating cancer cells to become less harmful—or even normal; by blocking the biological process that turns a normal cell into a cancerous one; and by enhancing the body's ability to repair normal cells that have been damaged by other types of cancer treatment such as chemotherapy and radiation therapy.

Slowly but surely, scientists are having success with these extremely difficult and arcane processes. Much of biological therapy is still in the investigational stage, but the Food and Drug Administration has approved treatments for some cancers, such as interferon alpha for hairy cell leukemia and Kaposi's sarcoma. And in fall 1998, a genetically engineered agent called Herceptin was approved treatment of metastatic breast cancer. (In biological therapy they're called *agents*, not *drugs*, because they are not chemicals, and the agents are sometimes called *biological response modifiers*.) There is no doubt that biological therapy will be an important tool for treating cancer; eventually it will probably become even more important than chemotherapy.

How the Immune System Works

If you remember from Chapter 1, a theory of the causation of cancer holds that the immune system has become defective, which results in a condition called *immunosuppression* or *immunodeficiency* (scientists sometimes refer to the system as *immunocompromised*). This requires some explanation; most people have heard of the immune system but are not quite sure how it works.

The immune system consists of a number of cells that act in concert to recognize, fight, and destroy foreign substances (*antigens*) that enter the body. They act the same way against an abnormally dividing cell or group of cells, which are perceived by the body as foreign substances. This is known as the *immune response*. The major cell components are these:

> ➤ *Macrophages* are the first line of defense. These cells recognize and engulf antigens, break them down into smaller components, and turn them over to T-lymphocytes. Macrophages produce substances called *cytokines*, which regulate the activity of lymphocytes.

➤ B-lymphocytes (also called *B-cells*) produce *antibodies*, which are proteins that recognize antigens and other foreign substances and attach themselves to them.
➤ T-lymphocytes (*T-cells*) are cells that recognize, respond to, and remember antigens. They manufacture *lymphokines*, which are substances that signal other cells. T-cells can destroy cancer cells on contact. Helper or suppressor T-cells stimulate or inhibit antibody production.
➤ *Polymorphonuclear leukocytes* is the general name for a group of white blood cells—neutrophils, basophils, and eosinophils—which were described in Chapter 3. Neutrophils are the most common and are the major constituent of pus because their main function is to fight infection. Basophils and eosinophils contain large granules, or storage sacs, and they interact with certain foreign materials.

The actions of these cells form a coordinated effort. In order to create and maintain this "teamwork," the cells must communicate with one another. They do this by secreting a number of different cytokines:

➤ *Interleukins* 1 through 12 (interleukin-2 has been effective in treating malignant melanoma and kidney cancer, although it has serious adverse effects)
➤ *Interferons* alpha (useful in hairy cell leukemia), beta, and gamma
➤ *Tumor necrosis factors* (TNF) alpha and beta
➤ *Prostaglandins*, substances that are active in tissue biochemistry

All these terms probably sound like Greek to you, and unless you're a molecular biologist, there's no reason why they shouldn't. Neither is there is reason why you need to commit them to memory, but they are included here in case your oncologist recommends biological therapy to you, and you begin to hear a lot of new vocabulary. If this happens, you at least have a reference to turn to if your doctor starts throwing these words around.

Anti-tumor Immunity

When the immune system recognizes a foreign substance (called an *antigen*), one of two responses ensues. In the *humoral response*, B-lymphocytes attach to the antigen, which in turn creates plasma cells that produce antibodies against the antigen. In the *cell-mediated response*, T-lymphocytes recognize the antigen and either kill it directly or elicit production of antibodies from plasma cells. Regulation of T-cell production and activity is controlled by cytokines, such as interleukin-1 and interleukin-2, and tumor necrosis factor, a natural protein produced by the body that may cause tumors to shrink.

In terms of malignancy, there is a concept known as *natural immunity* (also called *immune surveillance*), which holds that the immune system can recognize all tumor cells as foreign. This immunity is conferred by *natural killer cells* (a type of lymphocyte) and macrophages. This mechanism is not yet fully understood and obviously the system is not foolproof (if it were foolproof, we would not fall victim to the disease), perhaps because not all human tumors elicit such a response, or they are not sufficiently sensitive to the effects of killer cells.

Nevertheless, there has been some research on these cells that has resulted in *anti-tumor* therapies, several of which are now being tested in humans, some of which will be described later in the chapter.

Vaccine Therapy

One type of cancer appears to respond to vaccine therapy—and if there is one now, more will follow in the near future. Scientists observed that the immune system seems to play an important role in malignant melanoma, a virulent type of cancer that is often quickly fatal. These observations include: natural waxing and waning of melanoma lesions; the highly variable rate of disease progression; the possibility of late relapse; the increased incidence of the disease in immunosuppressed people; and the therapeutic efficacy of interleukin-2, which has its anti-tumor effect on the immune system.

Early attempts to develop a vaccine against melanoma were mostly unsuccessful, but modern molecular biology has led to the discovery of a large number of melanoma-associated antigens

(MAAs) that can induce an immune response in patients with the disease.

Because MAAs are weak antigens, melanoma patients need to be immunized repeatedly for prolonged periods, and sometimes the efficacy of the vaccine is enhanced by administering another vaccine called *bacillus Calmette-Guerin* (BCG), or drugs that affect the immune system such as cyclophosphamide, cimetadine, or indomethacin. These drugs have been found to help counteract the immunosuppression induced by the tumor.

In general, most cancer vaccines are therapeutic rather than prophylactic (that is, they treat a disease rather than prevent it), and they are made from attenuated cells or parts of cells. The theory behind immunotherapy with cancer vaccines is that they stimulate the patient's immune system to destroy tumor cells and thereby overcome the immunosuppression caused by factors related to the tumor. Vaccine therapy also attempts to enhance the ability of tumor-associated antigens (proteins possibly produced by the tumor) to stimulate a healthy immune response.

Chemotherapeutic drugs kill cells immediately, but cancer vaccines have no direct cytotoxic effect on existing disease. Rather, they elicit immune responses that require 12 to 14 weeks to take effect and perhaps six to eight months to induce complete remission. After the initial immunization, it takes about four to eight weeks for the growth rate of the tumor to slow; then there is a period of tumor stability and finally signs of regression.

Genes and Cancer

Again, if you're like most people, you know that genes exist, and you know they have something to do with heredity, but beyond that, things are a bit of a blur. And it may be news to you that genes are connected with cancer. (Don't feel bad. It was *big* news to the scientists who discovered the links between cancer and genetics.)

Genes are the physical units of heredity, and they can be defined as segments of genetic material that determine the sequence of *amino acids* (the substance of which proteins are made). Amino acids are found in certain chemicals called *polypeptides*, which are compounds composed of two or more amino acids. All of this is a fancy way of saying that these are the proteins of which much of your flesh is made.

Genes are composed of nucleic acids. In viruses, they are called *ribonucleic acid* (RNA), and in all other animal life, they are *deoxyribonucleic acid* (DNA). They are located within the chromosomes of every living cell.

Although the number of nucleic acids in genes is not infinite, it might as well be for their great numbers and the complexity with which they are arranged in patterns (the double helix with which you may be familiar). However, scientists are beginning to learn and understand the pattern, and in fact, in the United States, this decoding process is a major scientific endeavor. It is called the Human Genome Project, a combined project of the National Institutes of Health and private institutions. It will cost taxpayers billions of dollars by the time the decoding process is complete. But it's money well spent if it results in finding the cause of some cancers.

Genes that cause the growth of tumors (oncogenes) and those that prevent cancer cell growth (tumor suppressor genes) have recently been discovered—one of the greatest scientific discoveries of all time. Research on molecular mechanisms that control cell growth, differentiation, and proliferation also has led to a greater understanding of the nature of cancer.

Moreover, discovery of a series of genes responsible for many types of hereditary cancers will make it possible to screen people from families with a high incidence of cancer and other risk factors. Researchers also have found that a certain gene, called p53, when damaged or not present, can result in a cell becoming cancerous. This gene, p53, may be responsible for 60 percent of all cancers.

Genetics

Genetics is the branch of biology that deals with heredity, the attempt to explain similarities and differences that exist between parents and their offspring. Genetics has become an important part of the study of cancer because so many types of the disease are familial, and some, such as breast and colorectal cancer, may even be hereditary. Therefore, if one can understand the mechanism of how cancer is transmitted from generation to generation, one might be able to find the gene or genes responsible.

In fact, this is already beginning to happen. Scientists have recently discovered that some normal genes are transformed into genes that promote the development of cancer. These are the onco-genes described in Chapter 1.

Biological Therapy

New classes of anti-tumor agents have been discovered, including monoclonal antibodies and growth regulatory factors, which show promise in cancer treatment. There is now some evidence that resist-ance to chemotherapeutic drugs is due to biological changes in cancer cells, and recent clinical trials have shown that these changes can be manipulated to re-establish the sensitivity of tumor cells to drugs.

Immunotherapy

A fundamental theory in immunotherapy is that the immune system can help destroy cancer cells. The major problem with this approach is that the immune system may not recognize cancer cells as foreign because the difference between a tumor cell and a normal cell can be insignificant. However, if immunotherapy does work—and it often does not—it does so in one of several ways.

> *Active stimulation* is based on the theory that all humans beings have at least some anti-tumor immunity, and if these natural defenses can be stimulated, they can fight off cancer cells.
> *Adoptive therapy* involves transplanting immune cells or mol-ecules that carry lymphokines to increase the efficacy of the entire system.
> *Restorative therapy* replaces cells of the immune system destroyed by the cancer, chemotherapy, and other treatment modalities.
> *Passive therapy* means giving the immune system weapons such as antibodies or anti-tumor factors that can attack spe-cific cells.
> *Tumor cell modulation* heightens immune cells' ability to rec-ognize certain antigens on the surface of cancer cells.

Antibody Therapy

Antibody therapy uses monoclonal antibodies to seek and destroy cancer cells. *Monoclonal antibodies* (MAbs) are produced in a laboratory from one parent cell. Each antibody contains only the specific genetic material of the parent cell, which thus responds to only one specific antigen. MAbs are cloned cells. Uses for MAbs include:

➤ Bone marrow transplantation to kill cancer cells in bone marrow that has been removed from cancer patients. Unfortunately, antigens in cancer cells can develop resistance to monoclonal antibodies. See Chapter 5 for a description of how bone marrow transplantation works.

➤ Attaching them to chemotherapeutic drugs by means of a chemical bond. This allows the drugs to home in directly on specific cancer cells—and only on those cells. This minimizes many of the drugs' toxic effects.

➤ Programming them to carry a radioisotope to a tumor where the radioactive particles destroy malignant cells.

A monoclonal antibody, which is manufactured in a laboratory, is a specific antibody that can locate and attach to a specific protein, in this case one on a cancer cell. This means that a single antibody can be reproduced indefinitely in great quantities for relatively low cost. Not only can monoclonals be used to treat the disease, but they also can be used to diagnose cancer. For diagnosis purposes, they are made radioactive and injected into the bloodstream, where they home in on cancer cells. They then can be detected by sensing devices.

Herceptin, the agent mentioned earlier, is a monoclonal antibody that inhibits the growth of tumor cells. It is indicated for treatment of patients with metastatic breast cancer who have tumors that secrete too much of the gene called HER-2 (human epithelial growth factor receptor-2). The agent was developed at Genentech, Inc, a biotechnology company, because breast cancer patients who have too much HER-2 have a particularly poor prognosis and significantly decreased survival. The gene makes the cancer spread particularly aggressively in this group of women, which comprises about 25 to 30 percent of all breast cancer patients.

The HER-2 gene is involved in replication of many types of cells. However, when the gene is present in extra numbers, and as a result is overexpressed in breast or ovarian cancer cells, those cells replicate out of control. HER-2 produces a specific protein on cell surfaces, where it receives signals from outside the cell and relays them to the nucleus, directing the cell to replicate. In a cell that overproduces the HER-2 protein, Herceptin binds to the protein, thus preventing the cell from receiving and/or transmitting the growth stimulatory signal that would tell it to replicate.

Herceptin is the first successful cancer treatment that targets a specific genetic alteration without attacking healthy cells, and the first genetically engineered agent for treatment of metastatic breast cancer. Therefore, it avoids many of the serious side effects associated with traditional chemotherapy, including hair loss.

Gene Therapy

Scientists are now in the process of trying to work out a way to deliver certain genetic information to stem cells and tumor cells. If genes that are resistant to cancer (and other diseases) could be inserted into stem cells or tumor cells, the cells might "inherit" this resistance to cancer—and would not turn malignant. In tumor cells, the genetic information could be used to convert malignant cells to normal ones.

Gene therapy was first used on a human patient in 1990, and on a cancer patient the next year. It is still in early stages of development, but it is a definite reality. It will soon be used to develop drugs that block certain proteins that control chemical codes within cells' DNA, thereby "shutting out" genes that control malignant cell division.

There are a number of major fields of investigation in genetic therapy. One involves blocking a particular oncogene called *ras*, which turns cells cancerous. In addition, there is evidence that eradication or mutation of the p53 tumor suppressor gene is associated with tumor growth and progression. Therefore, manipulation of the normal gene, which can now be accomplished in animals, results in tumor inhibition. In other words, altering expression of the gene can be therapeutically beneficial.

Another area of investigation is transfusion with cancer-killing cells called tumor-infiltrating lymphocytes (TIL), which are taken from a patient's own cancerous tumor. When cancer occurs in the body, TIL cells occur naturally and migrate to the site of the cancer, where they invade the tumor. TIL cells also travel to cancer cells that have broken off from the tumor and spread elsewhere. This sounds as if it would be the perfect solution to the presence of cancer: the body doing the job on its own. Unfortunately, it's not possible to naturally manufacture sufficient TIL cells to destroy the entire tumor. So scientists extract TIL cells from the patient, enhance them with a gene capable of producing an anti-tumor substance (called tumor necrosis factor), and then transfuse them back into the patient, where they naturally migrate to the tumor.

Biological Agents Used in Cancer Therapy

Blood Growth Factors

Blood growth factors, also called *hematopoietic* growth factors or *colony-stimulating factors*, stimulate production of various cells in the blood. Growth factors are a family of cytokines that interact with specific receptors on hematopoietic cells (those that eventually develop into blood cells). They regulate the function of cells, and now with the development of recombinant DNA technology, it is possible to synthesize and manufacture pharmacologic doses of hematopoietic growth factors.

Most conventional combination chemotherapy regimens have dose-limiting toxicities that create limitations on how much of a drug or combination can be given safely. Most of these serious toxicities center on blood components. For example, *neutropenia* (abnormally low number of neutrophils) and *thrombocytopenia* (abnormally low platelet level) place patients at risk for serious, even life-threatening, infections and bleeding disorders.

Current clinical research centers around two major areas of hematopoietic growth factors: how to administer them appropriately in order to facilitate more dose-intense chemotherapy, and use of growth factors for supportive therapy to manage or decrease complications of chemotherapy.

There are now a limited number of randomized trials that, despite having only a few patients, are providing evidence to support the use of growth factors along with chemotherapy in certain situations.

Erythropoietin

Recombinant human *erythropoietin* (EPO), a factor that stimulates production of red cells, can differentiate stem cells from one lineage to another (remember that stem cells are the precursors of all blood cells). Many cancer patients have low red cell levels, and the lower the level, the more severe their anemia. It thus makes sense to give cancer patients EPO, and in early randomized studies with placebo controls, researchers demonstrated a statistically significant difference between patients receiving chemotherapy with supplemental EPO and those who were not given EPO. Later open-label, non-randomized trials with about 3,000 patients confirmed the benefits of EPO, both in terms of how the patients felt and the way their tumors responded. (See Chapter 6 for a discussion of how clinical trials are conducted.) EPO significantly increased hemoglobin levels, and it did it with all types of cancer (but not in all patients) and regardless of the type of chemotherapy used. Scientists speculate that the response is so universal because bone marrow mechanisms are the same in everyone.

EPO therapy is controversial though. There is solid evidence from randomized clinical trials that support the safety and efficacy of EPO, as well as non-randomized trials that prove quality-of-life benefits. But physicians cannot predict the types of patients who will benefit from EPO, and there are concerns about the high cost of a drug (about $1,200 per month) that does not save lives. In other words, how much is it worth for patients to feel better and function better, and will the high cost of the drug be offset by economic benefits such as getting cancer patients back to work?

Thrombopoietin

Another such biologic agent is *thrombopoietic growth factor* (also called *thrombopoietin*), which fights thrombocytopenia (dangerously low platelet count), a common serious side effect of chemotherapy. Thrombopoietic growth factors are useful in preventing bleeding that occurs due to an insufficient number of platelets, and they reduce the number and frequency of platelet transfusions. (There are about 8 million platelet transfusions in the United States each year, most of them for cancer patients.) In addition, they can be used to increase or maintain chemotherapy dosing regimens—because patients don't have to be withdrawn from chemotherapy or have the dose reduced because they are bleeding.

There is very little acute toxicity associated with thrombopoietin. This has led to trials of patients and normal volunteers to see if the efficiency of platelet collection from blood donors can be enhanced. In general, platelet production and yield were increased by about three-fold, and patients who were given these platelets experienced a four-fold increase in platelet counts.

Colony-Stimulating Factors

Colony-stimulating factors (CSF) are not anti-tumor agents, but they increase the number and activity of neutrophils and/or macrophages, which has increased the safety of high-dose chemotherapy for solid tumors, myeloma, lymphomas (including Hodgkin's disease), leukemia, and non-small cell lung cancer. They do not save lives, and they are very expensive.

CSFs reduce the risk of febrile (accompanied by a fever) neutropenia by about 50 percent in patients receiving drugs that have a high risk of neutropenia, and they are especially useful in patients who have bone marrow failure, who have had prior radiotherapy, who have had an incidence of febrile neutropenia several years in the past, who have a poor performance status (generally not functioning well), and who have infections and wounds.

It is not now possible to predict febrile neutropenia and thus determine who might benefit from CSFs. There is a general feeling of which patients are at high risk for neutropenia (for example, those with a lymphocyte count of less than 700), but validating studies are needed.

CSFs are widely used during chemotherapy even though there is no definitive proof of their effect on quality of life. But they clearly do have great biologic potential, and physicians have a strong desire to use the most current therapy and to keep patients out of the hospital. Also, there are very few side effects. In addition, physicians suffer from a great fear of litigation and worry about what would happen if a patient who did not receive a growth factor died of infection. Some doctors think this is an unfounded fear, but the practice of "defensive medicine" is so widespread that agents that may or may not be useful are often given when they don't need to be—or when they probably won't work.

Granulocyte Colony-Stimulating Factor

The major biologic effect of *granulocyte colony-stimulating factor* (G–CSF) is to increase the function and survival of neutrophils, which decreases the chance of severe infection. The major side effect is bone pain.

A subset of this factor is *granulocyte-macrophage-colony-stimulating factor* (GM-CSF), which produces an increase in the production of mature neutrophils and macrophages. It sustains the viability and potentiates the function of neutrophils. It appears to increase the destruction of microbes as well.

Interleukins

Interleukins (IL) 1 through 12 are currently being tested to determine their use in cancer treatment. Interleukin-2 has been shown to increase the activity of lymphocytes, and interleukin-11 (marketed as Neumega) has a variety of biological activities, including increasing the platelet count.

IL-11 is currently being tested, and will probably be found useful, in two clinical scenarios: first and most important, in the secondary prevention of chemotherapy-induced thrombocytopenia (after a patient has required a transfusion), and second, in primary prevention when patients are given chemotherapy (especially doxorubicin and cyclophosphamide) in higher-than-standard doses.

The downside of IL-11 is that it is quite toxic: side effects include edema, headaches, pleural effusion (fluid in the lungs), and cardiac arrhythmias. But the toxicity needs to be balanced against the risk of transfer of viral agents (hepatitis and, rarely, AIDS) during transfusion.

Other Agents

A number of other biological agents have shown promise but are not yet as far down the research path as those just described. *Tumor necrosis factors*, also called lymphotoxins, stimulate immune cells, damage tumor cells directly, and make tumors more recognizable to the immune system. *Bacillus Calmette-Guerin* (BCG), a single-celled organism formerly used as a vaccine against tuberculosis, is now used to treat bladder cancer. Interferons, of which interferon alpha was the first cytokine to show an anti-tumor effect, originally had scientists optimistic but subsequently proved disappointing. They may, however, be useful when combined with cytotoxic drugs or other biological agents such as tumor necrosis factor or gamma interferon.

When to Use Biological Therapy

Biological therapy is still in very early stages of development, and although it has been used successfully on some patients for some cancers (malignant melanoma, breast cancer, kidney cancer, chronic myelogenous leukemia, and hairy cell leukemia), by and large it is still considered developmental, and almost all biological therapy is done as part of clinical trials.

In general, biological therapy is used when there is no standard treatment for a particular cancer or when the standard treatment has not been effective. This does not mean, however, that you should be afraid of biological therapy if your physician recommends it. You will not be a "guinea pig," and you will not be subjected to any more risks than you would with standard therapy.

Angiogenesis

One of the most exciting areas of cancer research is *angiogenesis*, the process by which tumors grow their own blood vessels, which then connect to the general circulatory system and through which tumor cells break off from the original site and travel to other parts of the body.

The pioneer in angiogenesis research is Judah Folkman, M.D., Director of the Surgical Research Laboratory at Children's Hospital in Boston. He recently announced that the process of angiogenesis is involved not only in solid tumors, as had been previously thought, but also in liquid or blood tumors. Dr. Folkman and his colleagues have discovered angiogenesis in the bone marrow of leukemia patients.

In the past decade, the study of angiogenesis and anti-angiogenic factors has leapt to the forefront of cancer research. Tumors cannot grow bigger than the size of a kernel of corn, says Dr. Folkman, unless they develop their own vasculature. Therefore, they lie dormant, undetected, and in situ (and thus relatively harmless) until something triggers them to secrete growth factors that induce the formation of new blood vessels. Once a tumor is angiogenic, it is potentially fatal. The trick, then, is to find anti-angiogenic therapy.

The goal of such therapy is to disrupt the sequence of events that leads to angiogenesis and to halt, or even reverse, tumor growth. Several such agents are now being studied in laboratory animals, and others are already in clinical trials.

How Anti-Angiogenic Agents Work

Endothelial cells that line blood vessels produce substances called growth factors, more than a dozen of which have already been identified by scientists. Only tumor cells with receptors for a particular growth factor proliferate and thrive. Therefore, if the growth factor can be turned off—with anti-angiogenic agents (also called angiogenic inhibitors)—those tumor cells will die (in a process called apoptosis, which is a scientific way of saying that the cells commit suicide).

Dr. Folkman and other scientists believe that the best way to treat cancer is to target both types of cells simultaneously: cytotoxic agents to kill tumor cells, and angiogenic inhibitors to prevent endothelial cells from stimulating growth of the tumor. A major advantage of this "double whammy" treatment is that endothelial cells do not develop resistance to angiogenic inhibitors, whereas many cytotoxic agents eventually do induce drug resistance in tumor cells because they have a tendency to mutate, which means they are no longer the cells they originally were.

Two of the many promising angiogenic inhibitors that are now in clinical trials are angiostatin and endostatin, both naturally occurring proteins that are isolated from the very tumors that they are intended to treat. It will be several years before anti-angiogenic treatment is widely available—and that's only if the clinical trials prove that it works well.

Two other anti-angiogenic factors have been widely studied: interferon alpha and interferon beta. Interferons seem to inhibit RNA expression and protein production in some human carcinoma cells, especially renal, bladder, colon, and prostate cancer cells. It appears that interferon beta, which is produced by dividing cells, can regulate the process of angiogenesis, which is an integral part of the process of metastasis. Therefore, it might be used as a first line of defense against cancer.

Chapter Five

Bone Marrow Transplantation

A Potent Chemotherapeutic Treatment to Purge the Body of Cancer Cells

*B*one marrow transplantation (BMT) is the process of removing the bone marrow of a person with cancer, giving that person massive doses of chemotherapy to kill as many cancer cells as possible, and then transfusing healthy marrow from a donor back into the patient.

The theory behind this treatment is that in a patient with cancer, bone marrow, the production center for stem cells (which eventually mature into red and white blood cells and platelets) is defective, and if it can be replaced with normal tissue, the cancer will be defeated. This is an elegant theory—which doesn't always work in practice.

But often it does, and although bone marrow transplantation is an unpleasant and dangerous treatment, many people believe it is worth a try—for two major reasons. First, transplanted marrow can act directly on a cancer like leukemia because the patient is actually receiving the immune system of another person—the donor. This transplanted immune system then can recognize the patient's own cancer cells as foreign and abnormal and destroy them.

Second, BMT is used to support other chemotherapy and radiation therapy. Because bone marrow is the tissue most sensitive to the effects of chemotherapy and radiation, if those treatments are given in high enough doses to kill tumor cells (called high-dose chemotherapy, an increasingly common approach to cancer treatment), there is a good chance that it will also kill stem cells in the marrow. So if the marrow can be replaced with healthy donor marrow after the course of high-dose chemotherapy or radiation, those treatments could be given in sufficient therapeutic doses to kill tumor cells without having to worry about the toxic effects on stem cells. Using BMT in this way can mean the difference between *palliation* (reduction of symptoms and improvement of quality of life without hope of cure) and cure.

Third, transplantation of allogeneic marrow (that of another person) provides an anti-tumor effect that is separate from that conferred by chemotherapy and/or radiation.

There are a number of reasons why BMT works so well, and in so many cases has cured cancer. First is the remarkable regenerative capacity of the tissue known as bone marrow. Transplantation of less than 10 percent of a donor's total body marrow can result in the complete and sustained replacement of the recipient's entire hematopoietic (blood production) system. After the transplant, the donated marrow produces all the recipient's red cells, most of the white cells, the platelets, as well as many other cellular components of blood.

Second, after transfusion of donated marrow (it is given intravenously, like a blood transfusion), it automatically homes in on the recipient's marrow space. No one knows why this happens, but without the marrow's ability to seek its home, BMT would not be possible.

Third, bone marrow can survive *cryopreservation* (freezing at supercold temperatures) with little, if any, damage. And the freezing technique used for BMT is relatively simple.

The first attempt at bone marrow transplantation was made in the 1930s, but it failed because the necessary highly specific tissue typing had not yet been discovered. Twenty years later, another attempt failed because techniques for freezing donated bone marrow were had not been perfected. Discovery of this typing in the 1960s made allogeneic transplantation a possibility. In the mid-1960s, successful transplants were done on dogs, and later that decade, the first successful transplants for treatment of leukemia were done in humans. During the following decade, BMT became an accepted, if not routine, part of treatment for certain cancers. With the advent of effective cryopreservation, BMT became widely available and remains so today—provided a compatible donor can be found.

By the 1970s, allogeneic BMT (from donated bone marrow) had become a generally accepted treatment, and in the late 1970s, autologous BMT (when the donor is oneself) was used to treat patients with lymphoma. It came into widespread use in the 1980s.

Between 1985 and 1990, the annual number of autologous BMTs in the United States increased by more than 600 percent—from less than 1,000 transplants per year to more than 6,000. During the same period, allogeneic transplants increased by 67 percent, from 3,000 to 5,000 each year. In the decade that followed, the rate of increase approximately doubled. The demand for BMT far outstrips the number performed because of the shortage of donors, but as of this writing, more than 15,000 people worldwide have undergone BMT.

BMT has been highly or moderately successful with many cancers: acute myeloid leukemia, acute lymphocytic leukemia, chronic myelogenous leukemia, chronic lymphocytic leukemia, hairy cell leukemia, Hodgkin's disease, non-Hodgkin's lymphomas, multiple myeloma, testicular cancer, neuroblastoma, and breast cancer (possibly).

Types of Transplants

Allogeneic Transplantation

Allogeneic BMT is transfer of marrow from one individual to another. The donor and recipient must be compatible for human leukocyte group A (HLA) antigens. Every single human being has genes on one particular chromosome that contain a code to recognize proteins on cell surfaces. These proteins (HLA antigens) are involved in cell self-recognition. Under a high-powered microscope, they can be individually identified, making it possible to compare bone marrow from one person to another. If the antigens are not compatible (matched), the patient's bone marrow will attack that of the donor, and it will be rejected.

The process is a little like biochemical fingerprinting. No two individuals have the same fingerprints—not even identical twins. Each and every fingerprint has its own distinctive pattern of whorls and loops that can be positively identified under a microscope, and unless yours are the on the gun that did the deed, you won't be found guilty. By the same token, if your HLAs don't closely match the donor's, the transplant won't be successful.

When bone marrow transplants were first performed, it was possible only between identical twins because the marrow would be genetically identical. Now it has been shown that if the marrow is very closely matched (ideally that which occurs between first-degree relatives) instead of perfectly matched, the transplant can be successful. In general, the better the match, the more successful the treatment.

Allogeneic transplantation can be done between two unrelated people, but it is difficult to find a compatible donor. HLA antigens are highly complex and consist of more than a billion combinations. However, it is not impossible, and with high-speed tissue analyzers, the National Marrow Donor Bank has been able to maintain records of people with the most common HLA antigens.

In terms of tissue matching, there has been recent good news from Japan. Researchers there have discovered that a more sophisticated matching system relies on DNA rather than HLA. They found that HLA antigens have a variety of subtypes that can be identified only by DNA testing, and the subtypes may be the most important factor in determining the success of the transplant—and the survival of the patient. Using DNA matching, which unfortunately adds to the complexity and expense of the pre-transplant procedure, could double the number of donors from whom a successful match could be made.

Syngeneic Transplantation

Syngeneic BMT occurs between identical twins. It carries the best likelihood of success, but the vast majority of cancer patients don't have a twin brother or sister.

Autologous Transplantation

Autologous BMT means that the same person is both donor and recipient. This seems paradoxical (even foolish when that person has cancer), but it has been done successfully. Bone marrow and/or peripheral blood (blood in the general circulation) is removed before chemotherapy and is stored by cryopreservation. When chemotherapy is complete, the marrow is returned to the patient. This eliminates the risk of rejection as well as graft versus host disease (see discussion of graft versus host disease that appears later in this chapter), but it creates a risk of reinfusing cancer cells that might possibly have been in the marrow. Some cancer centers are attempting to counter this risk by also subjecting the stored marrow to chemotherapy or irradiation. Other techniques to reduce the risk of reinfusing tumor cells include removing them by means of specially designed antibodies or immunomagnetic beads, and positive selection of normal stem cells—that is, picking out cells not contaminated by tumor.

Peripheral Stem Cell Transplantation

It is possible to collect stem cells for transplantation from the peripheral blood, the blood flowing through the circulatory system. A catheter is inserted through the skin and into a vein, usually in the chest just below the collarbone, and kept in place for a few weeks. This is done on an outpatient basis and requires only local anesthesia (in contrast to bone marrow harvesting, which is done under general anesthesia). Once the catheter is in place, the patient is connected to an *apheresis* machine. In this procedure, the blood flows into the machine, which separates the stem cells from the rest of the cells, which are then returned to the patient. This too is done on an outpatient basis—two or three times before the actual bone marrow transplant—and is similar to, but slightly more complex than, going to a blood donor center. It takes three or four hours, and the donor usually lies in an extremely comfortable reclining lounge chair instead of on a hard table.

Peripheral blood stem cell harvest may cause some dizziness and tingling in the hands and feet. Less common side effects include chills, tremors, and muscle cramps. They are all temporary and are caused by changes in the patient's blood volume as it circulates through the apheresis machine, as well as by blood thinners added to prevent clotting during the procedure.

One of the major disadvantages of peripheral stem cell transplantation is the low number of stem cells in the general circulation. This means that a huge volume of blood must be subjected to apheresis, which is expensive, uncomfortable, and not practical. On the plus side, however, more people are willing to donate peripheral stem cells than are willing to subject themselves to bone marrow donation.

Moreover, administration of hematopoietic growth factors— such as granulocyte colony-stimulating factor and granulocyte

macrophage colony-stimulating factor—has led to a marked increase
in the number of stem cells in the peripheral blood. Because of the
increasing ability to remove or kill tumor cells and the speed with
which growth factors are being developed (see Chapter 4), it is likely
that within the next decade or so, peripheral stem cell transplantation will replace bone marrow transplantation as the treatment of
choice for cancer.

After stem cells are collected by either process, they are taken to
the blood bank and frozen until it is time to reinfuse them.

Making the BMT Decision

Just as you would ask a surgeon, "Have you ever done this before?"
(or an electrician or a plumber, for that matter), if you need a bone
marrow transplant, you will need to find out where the most experienced transplant center is. Unless you are being treated at a major
cancer center, chances are your local hospital is not equipped to perform BMTs, and you'll have to travel out of town for the procedure.
There are some things you and your oncologist need to consider
when choosing a BMT center.

First, you will want to know how much experience the center
has had with BMT and what its track record is—that is, how successful it has been. You also should ask about the percentage of
patients who remain alive and disease free. By the way, don't be
afraid of asking about this. It is the single most important criterion
in measuring success of BMT, and the transplant center has the sta-
tistics and will give them to you if you ask.

You will also need to learn the minimum criteria required of a
cancer center in order to perform BMT; a list of the criteria is available from the American Society of Clinical Oncology and the
American Society of Hematology. Your health insurer has policies
about paying for BMT, and you have to know what they are before
embarking on the procedure. Find out by asking your insurance carrier or the billing personnel at the BMT center. BMT is very expensive, and the transplant center will want to know how and when it
will be paid before it will even consider taking care of you.

All BMT centers have policies about pretreatment tests and inter-
views. Find out what they are. In addition, you will need to ask

about the length of the waiting list at the center you have chosen, as well as the availability of a donor.

The Procedure

Adult bone marrow is found in the flat bones of the pelvis, ribs, spine, and collarbones (in children, it is found in all bones). It is removed from the donor, most often from the pelvic bones, by means of about 200 needle punctures. This is just as unpleasant and painful as it sounds, so the procedure is done under general anesthesia.

The way the marrow is handled after removal from the donor depends on the type of transplant. If it is allogeneic and if the donor and recipient have the same blood type, the marrow is given by intravenous injection to the recipient immediately. If the blood type of the donor and recipient are not compatible, the red blood cells are separated from the marrow and discarded. Then the marrow is given to the recipient. In an autologous transplant, the cells are frozen and stored.

An alternate method to collect stem cells is to separate them from the peripheral blood, the "regular bloodstream," in the procedure described earlier.

Peripheral stem cell transplant has one major advantage and one major disadvantage. It is not a surgical procedure, which makes it appeal to a much larger number of donors. On the other hand, there are far fewer stem cells in the peripheral blood than there are in the marrow, so a much greater volume of blood than of marrow is required for a transplant.

Reinfusion

When high-dose chemotherapy is complete, reinfusion begins. The process is similar to a blood transfusion, but instead of whole blood, frozen bags of bone marrow or stem cells are warmed in water and then injected through an indwelling catheter. The process takes three or four hours, during which the reinfused stem cells or marrow home in on the patient's own empty marrow space.

The most common side effects are caused by a preservative called dimethyl sulfoxide (DMSO), which was mixed with the bone marrow before cryopreservation. Problems include nausea and vomiting, abdominal cramps, chills, and a taste or odor of garlic. In rare instances, there might be hypotension (lowered blood pressure), tachycardia (fast heart rate), or shortness of breath. The side effects are temporary, and are easily relieved by medication.

Reinfused stem cells that have migrated to the marrow space take a few weeks to produce blood cells, in a process called *engraftment*. During that time, special precautions must be taken to prevent infection. You will be asked to have frequent checkups, so you'll need to stay near the treatment center. In some cases, patients will be hospitalized during the procedure and until engraftment is well established.

During the recovery period, you may need transfusions to replace red cells and platelets, medications to relieve lingering side effects of the high-dose chemotherapy, and intravenous fluids and nutrition if you are unable to eat. And as in all transplants, you will be given medications to prevent an allergic reaction to the new tissue. In addition, you will probably receive one or more types of colony-stimulating factors to encourage the engrafted stem cells to divide and mature into white cells as quickly as possible.

Serious efforts are made to prevent infection. You'll probably have to take antibiotics, and your visitors will be required to wear masks, gowns, and gloves to minimize contact. You won't be allowed to receive fresh flowers, plants, fruits, and vegetables because they tend to carry bacteria and fungi. Still, you won't have to subsist entirely on hospital food because your friends can bring "care packages" of any type of food that appeals to you.

Complications and Risks
Delayed Effects

High-dose chemotherapy or radiotherapy can cause cataracts, and massive exposure to irradiation can increase the risk of other cancers. Delayed effects also include sterility, although people who receive chemotherapy are often rendered sterile even without undergoing BMT. It is highly unlikely that you will contract AIDS from a BMT or from peripheral stem cells, or from the blood transfusions that follow, because blood is thoroughly tested for the AIDS virus. However, hepatitis B is an ever-present danger.

Immediate Effects
Drug Reactions

High-dose chemotherapy rarely (but not never) can cause deadly cardiac effects. Much more usual are the effects of chemotherapy (specifically cyclophosphamide) and radiation therapy: nausea and vomiting, mild skin erythema (redness), and oral mucositis, for which narcotic analgesia might be needed for a week or so.

High-dose chemotherapy can cause veno-occlusive disease of the liver in about 10 percent of patients. It is characterized by abdominal swelling and edema, tenderness, liver enlargement, and jaundice. About 30 percent of the patients who develop veno-occlusive disease of the liver will die of it.

Infection

Infection, most likely pneumonia, is one of the most common complications, because after the transplant, the new bone marrow takes about four to six weeks before it can produce red and white blood cells and platelets. Red cells and platelets can be replenished by transfusion, but white cells cannot. Therefore, the patient is highly vulnerable to infection—which, without sufficient white cells to fight it, can be fatal.

Pneumonia

The lungs seem to be particularly sensitive to the effects of BMT. Pneumonia can arise because of infection or as a result of high-dose chemotherapy. Either can cause death immediately after BMT or several months later.

Hemorrhage

Uncontrolled bleeding can occur as a result of a low platelet count. Sometimes the amount of platelets that can be replaced is insufficient to stop the bleeding.

Fatigue and Difficulty Breathing

Lack of red blood cells that carry oxygen can cause fatigue, a common symptom of anemia, and difficulty breathing. Red blood cells replenish themselves quickly, so these problems are short-lived. If they persist, you might be given a transfusion of red cells.

Graft Rejection

This risk increases in significance as the number of unmatched antigens increases. Marrow function appears to regenerate but then ceases, or it never returns at all. The patient's immune system perceives the new marrow as foreign and attacks it. Graft failure after autologous transplant usually results from marrow damage between the time it was removed from the patient and the time it was reinfused, what doctors call ex vivo treatment. A second transplant can be attempted but from a different donor.

Graft Versus Host Disease

Sometimes the allogeneic graft (transplanted tissue of any type, not just bone marrow) goes "overboard," and its white blood cells recognize the host's (yours) normal tissue as abnormal and thus attacks and kills more than just cancer cells.

The condition is uncommon, but when it happens, it occurs any time between nine days and a year after transplant (but usually within three months) and affects people whose immune system is compromised by drugs or disease. Graft versus host disease (GVHD) most often affects the skin (rash, especially on the palms and soles of the feet), liver (abnormal changes in liver enzymes), and gastrointestinal system (loss of appetite and diarrhea), and usually can be prevented and/or treated. Other symptoms include fever, low blood pressure, destruction of tissue, and shock.

Prevention of GVHD begins with pretreatment with a combination of cyclosporine and methotrexate or another immunosuppressive drug, as well as prednisone, that you also will take for many months after the transplant.

The Future of BMT

A number of factors ensures that BMT has a promising future in a wider variety of cancers :

> ➤ Its use in leukemias and lymphomas has already become fairly standard, and more patients with carcinomas and sarcomas will benefit from BMT—and may even be cured.

➤ Hematopoietic growth factors can accelerate growth of bone marrow after transplantation, thus decreasing the risk of infection that accompanies BMT.

➤ Greater use will be made of peripheral blood stem cell collection for transplantation, thus increasing the number of patients who are candidates for autologous transplantation.

➤ The National Marrow Donor Program has a huge computerized database to identify unrelated potential donors, which also increases the number of people who can undergo BMT.

➤ The safety of BMT will be improved as advances are made in the prevention and treatment of post-transplant infections.

➤ The most important area of future research involves ways to eradicate the underlying malignancy. High-dose chemotherapy combined with BMT has proved effective, but there is a significant risk of serious toxicity, even death, from the drugs themselves. Scientists are now looking at ways to use monoclonal antibodies or other agents that can carry even higher doses of chemotherapy or radiotherapy directly to tumor cells.

Chapter Six

Clinical Trials

How New Treatments are Developed and How They Can Benefit Your Recovery

A clinical trial is the process by which a new drug is tested in humans, or by which an existing FDA-approved drug is tested for a new use (called an *indication*). It is a scientific study designed to answer questions about the actions and safety of chemotherapeutic and biological agents. The drug being tested is considered *investigational* (*not* experimental). The process of clinical trials is required by the Food and Drug Administration before any drug or medical device can be manufactured, prescribed, and sold to the public.

Clinical trials are the *only* scientific mechanism to test the safety and efficacy of drugs—all drugs, not just those used to treat cancer. This type of research is the foundation on which all accepted medical practice is based, and the likelihood of discovering new and effective cancer treatments without clinical trials is minuscule.

Wait! Back up a minute. "Tested in humans." Does this mean you? Quite possibly, yes. But before you start walking backward, saying, "Whoa, I'm no guinea pig," and before you learn about how clinical trials are conducted, look at the many advantages:

> ➤ New drugs may be more effective than standard drugs, especially if standard treatment didn't work for you. Or an already approved drug for one type of cancer may be found to work in another type (yours, for instance), but FDA reg-

ulations require that it go through the same process as when it was first approved. This is a very common occurrence.

➤ Clinical trials are conducted under extremely strict conditions (called a *protocol*), and there are more safety checks in operation than when a physician prescribes standard therapy.

➤ Because you are required to sign a consent form, you will have complete information about the drug: all its effects and all its side effects—probably much more than you wanted to know.

➤ You're the "first kid on the block" to have access to a new and most likely beneficial treatment.

➤ Your risk of harm or injury is minimal because there are stringent federal laws and regulations in place to protect clinical trials subjects. In fact, the risks are much *lower* than they are with standard therapy.

➤ The drug has been thoroughly tested in the laboratory, on animals—and on other people long before you volunteer for the trial—so you are not taking a drug about which little or nothing is known.

➤ The treatment is free—and many insurance companies and HMOs are now willing to pay for the ancillary care—that is, the cost of hospitalization if it's necessary, as well as the cost of administering the drug.

➤ You are doing a tremendous service to medical science—and to yourself.

Purpose of Clinical Trials

The purpose of clinical trials is to determine *safety* and *efficacy*. Every advance in all of American medicine, and particularly oncology, since the early part of this century has been as a result of clinical trials. In fact, it is impossible (and illegal) to approve a new drug or treatment without them. If your physician suggests that you enter a clinical trial, consider it seriously.

It is a popular belief that a clinical trial represents a last-ditch effort, that if you participate in one then you must be at death's door. *This is not true.* Today, clinical trials are carefully controlled studies in which the subjects (patients or healthy volunteers) know exactly what is happening every step of the way. They are told all about the drug to be tested, as well as its risks and known side effects. What's more, any subject can withdraw from the trial at any time and for any reason.

Types of Clinical Trials

There are two basic types of clinical trials: *randomized, double blind;* and *open label*. In the former, no one knows who is taking the drug under investigation and who is taking the standard therapy. The group of subjects is randomly assigned to one of these two subgroups, also called *arms* (the one taking the other therapy is called the *control group*). Neither the investigators nor the subjects have a clue, and the codes under which the drugs are assigned to the two groups of subjects are not broken until the study is finished.

In open label, everyone knows who is taking which agent. Although a randomized, double blind trial is considered more scientifically valid, there are legitimate reasons for doing an open label study, such as if a drug is being compared to radiation, or if one arm of the trial is surgery plus a drug and the other is surgery alone.

Clinical Protocol

A clinical protocol is an extremely detailed written description of a treatment program, in this case, a description of the drug under investigation and the conditions under which the trial is to be conducted. Included in the protocol are the purpose of the investigation; the nature of the drug or treatment under investigation; anticipated outcomes (what the investigators think the drug will do—that is, how it will behave in the body); risks to patients; criteria for participation in the trial; and the methods used to monitor safety and check for adverse effects.

Every medical institution that conducts clinical trials has an Institutional Review Board (IRB)—also known as a Human Use Committee—composed of physicians and scientists who have no relationship with the physicians conducting the clinical trial. The purpose of the IRB is to protect the rights of the human subjects, and no clinical trial may take place without IRB approval. In a reputable institution, the criteria for allowing a trial to go forward are *very* rigorous. If the institution receives federal funds (and it's almost impossible for medical research to be conducted without them), then the clinical trials also are overseen by the National Institutes of Health—in the case of oncology drugs, the National Cancer Institute.

An Actual Clinical Trial

The Breast Cancer Prevention Trial (BCPT) was a clinical trial designed to determine whether taking the drug tamoxifen (manufactured under the trade name Nolvadex) could lower the chance of breast cancer in women who are at high risk of developing the disease. The BCPT also looked at whether taking tamoxifen decreased the number of heart attacks and reduced the number of bone fractures in these women.

Tamoxifen is an oral hormonal agent that had been used for 25 years to treat advanced breast cancer, and for the past 15 years as adjuvant therapy following surgery and/or radiation for early-stage breast cancer. The drug works, in part, by interfering with the activity of estrogen, a female hormone that promotes growth of breast cancer cells.

In a stroke of serendipity, researchers came to realize that adjuvant tamoxifen therapy does two things: it prevents the original breast cancer from returning, and it helps prevent development of new cancers in the same or opposite breast. Therefore, they postulated, tamoxifen might have a similar beneficial effect for women at increased risk of the disease, especially those whose first-degree female relatives (mother, sister, daughter) had breast cancer. Moreover, while tamoxifen acts *against* the effects of estrogen in breast tissue, it acts *like* estrogen in other body systems. Hence, it could lower blood cholesterol and slow bone loss.

The study began recruiting participants in April 1992 and closed enrollment in September 1997; 13,388 women were enrolled. Women aged 60 and older qualified to participate on the basis of age alone (the risk of breast cancer increases with age), and women aged 35 to 59 participated if they were at an increased risk of breast cancer. The study was conducted at more than 300 medical centers in the United States and Canada by researchers with the National Surgical Adjuvant Breast and Bowel Project (NSABP), one of the most prestigious groups of cancer researchers in the world. It was funded by the National Cancer Institute.

Participants in the randomized, double blind BCPT received either tamoxifen or a placebo (an inert substance), and risk for women under age 60 was assessed by means of the following criteria: number of first-degree relatives who had been diagnosed with the disease; age at delivery of a woman's first child; the number of times she had undergone a breast biopsy, especially if she had had atypical hyperplasia (oftentimes a precursor to cancer); and age at first menstrual period.

Women were not allowed to participate in the BCPT if they were at high risk of developing blood clots, and/or if they were taking hormone replacement therapy or oral contraceptives (unless they stopped taking these medications three months prior to entering the study). Women also were disqualified if they were pregnant or planned to become pregnant during the five years they would be on the study because animal studies suggested that tamoxifen might be teratogenic (causing fetal malformations).

In the trial, healthy women assigned to take tamoxifen developed 85 cases of invasive breast cancer compared with 154 cases in the women taking the placebo.

However, tamoxifen did increase the women's chances of acquiring three rare but life-threatening health problems: there were 33 cases of endometrial cancer in the tamoxifen group versus 14 in the placebo group, although it was not associated with any other type of cancer; there were 17 cases of pulmonary embolism (blood clot in the lung) in the tamoxifen group compared with 6 cases among women taking the placebo; and there were 30 cases of deep vein thrombosis (blood clots in major veins) in women who took tamoxifen and 19 cases in the placebo group.

Some women in both groups experienced minor side effects: vaginal dryness, itching, or bleeding; menstrual irregularities; depression; loss of appetite; nausea and/or vomiting; dizziness; headache; and fatigue. The major side effects experienced by women in the tamoxifen group were hot flashes and vaginal discharge.

While tamoxifen is not without some danger in and of itself, its benefits clearly outweigh the risks, and on the basis of the trial results, in September 1998 the FDA approved tamoxifen for breast cancer risk reduction. As of this writing, the recommendation is for women to take tamoxifen for only five years. In a related study, women with early-stage breast cancer who took tamoxifen for five years showed no greater benefit than did women who took it for ten years—and those who took the drug for longer periods of time tended to have more adverse effects.

So—if you are at high risk of breast cancer or have already had it, should you take tamoxifen? As with any other chemotherapy, you need to discuss this with your physicians, but it seems that for the vast majority of high-risk women, the benefits outweigh the risks.

The BCPT is fully enrolled, which means the researchers have all the subjects they need, but the NSABP will conduct other breast cancer risk reduction trials. If you are interested in finding out more about future plans, contact them on the Internet at *www.nsabp.pitt.edu* or by mail at NSABP, Box 21, Pittsburgh, PA 15261. The fax number is (412) 330-4664. To find out about participation in other clinical trials, see the following sections.

Pharmaceutical Manufacture and Control

Although you may not be interested in the details of pharmaceutical manufacturing, a brief outline of the process is included here because for the next year or two, your life is going to be pretty much ruled by drugs—powerful and complex ones. These drugs have been manufactured to kill a powerful and complex disease, and their discovery and production has taken millions of hours of scientific effort and billions of dollars in both public and private money. Therefore, it stands to reason that you might be curious about the substances flowing into your veins.

In the United States, except for about half of all cancer drugs, most drug development and manufacturing is done by pharmaceutical companies. The other half are developed by researchers associated with institutions like the National Cancer Institute and universities. A recent survey conducted by the American Society of Clinical Oncology found that to a greater and greater extent, investigators themselves must subsidize clinical trials because funding from traditional sources (the federal government and the private sector) is shrinking.

The FDA, a division of the U.S. Public Health Service, Department of Health and Human Services, does not develop drugs, and it does not test them. It is, however, required by law to ensure that all drugs manufactured and sold in the United States are safe and effective.

The FDA was established in 1906 with the passage of the Food and Drug Act, which prohibited interstate commerce in misbranded and adulterated food, drinks, and drugs. This was the first federal effort to get rid of "snake oil medicine" and protect consumers from the thousands of purveyors of highly unsafe food and drugs, many of which were toxic. Since that time, the FDA's range of legal and administrative functions has expanded enormously, but the one of primary concern to you now is guaranteeing efficacy and safety.

The FDA has many divisions and departments, but the two most pertinent to this discussion is the Center for Drug Evaluation Research and the Center for Biologics Research. These are the people who decide which drugs and biologicals are approved for sale in the United States and which are not.

The process takes an incredibly long time, costs hundreds of millions of dollars (mostly of private money), and is extremely complex and often frustrating—for the pharmaceutical company. For consumers, the complexity of the approval process and the number of safeguards built into it should be very reassuring. Here is a thumbnail sketch of how a drug is discovered, developed, tested, and approved.

First, a compound is isolated in a laboratory or discovered in nature and is subjected to testing to see if it has a pharmacologic effect. This is done in test tubes and with other laboratory apparatus (in vitro), by computer, or in animals (in vivo). During this stage, toxicologists look for potentially harmful or fatal effects of the substance, pharmacologists analyze how the agent works in the body, and computer scientists analyze and assess the drug's properties. This first phase is called preclinical evaluation.

If the agent does indeed have an effect and if it is thought that it will be effective and safe for human use, clinical trials are begun. Clinical trials are human tests and consist of three phases.

> ➤ Phase I, the main purpose of which is safety (to establish the maximum tolerated dose) and toxicity, involves 20 to 200 people and lasts several months. About 70 percent of all drugs make it through this phase. With non-cancer drugs, sometimes normal volunteers are used in Phase I, but in oncology, actual patients participate in Phase I, and the intent is therapeutic. This is the only type of clinical trial in which a drug has not yet been tested in humans.

> Phase II, which looks again at safety but is mainly concerned with efficacy (anti-tumor activity) and dose response (the way patients respond to a drug at various dose levels), involves several hundred people and lasts several months to two or three years. Most clinical investigators prefer patients who have not yet been treated for cancer (in medical parlance, they're called *treatment naïve*) or who have received little or no benefit from previous treatment. About 33 percent of the drugs that made it through Phase I pass successfully through Phase II trials.

> Phase III, which is concerned with safety, efficacy, and regulation of dosage, involves several hundred to several thousand people and lasts one to four years. It is usually the trial that defines the role of a particular drug in a chemotherapy regimen—that is, whether it is best used alone or in combination. The drug under consideration is either compared with another drug or is used in combination with one or more other drugs. Researchers look at the following parameters as compared with heretofore standard treatment: effect on survival, rate and duration of response, toxicity, and quality of life improvement. Only about 25 percent of successful Phase II drugs make it through Phase III.

When the clinical trials are finished, the pharmaceutical manufacturer formally asks for FDA approval. The FDA has been aware of and involved in the entire process, because at each step of the way, the manufacturer must secure FDA approval for the next step.

The manufacturer then presents its findings at a meeting of an FDA drug advisory committee. In the case of cancer drugs it's the Oncologic Drugs Advisory Committee, which is composed of private individuals—usually physicians and other scientists who are leaders in their respective fields. The committee meetings take place in suburban Washington, D.C. and are open to the public.

Once in a while, an investigational drug will be given to a patient or small group of patients who have not participated in any of the clinical trials for that drug on what is called a *compassionate basis*. This occurs when all standard treatments for those patients have failed, when the new drug has passed through Phase II or Phase III trials, and when a licensed physician requests and makes a good case for compassionate use. The request is made to the pharmaceutical company, which is not allowed to charge for compassionate use.

Before the advisory committee is convened, an army of FDA scientists goes over all the data about the drug submitted by the manufacturer. Chemists focus on how the drug is made, and whether the manufacturing, control, and packaging are adequate. Pharmacologists evaluate the effects of the drug on animals and humans. Physicians look at the results of the clinical trials, including beneficial and adverse effects, and whether the proposed labeling (directions to physicians about how to use the drug) accurately reflect its effects. Pharmacokineticists measure the rate and extent to which the drug's active ingredient is made available to the body and how it is metabolized and eliminated. Statisticians determine if the animal studies and clinical trials were well designed, well controlled, and accurately reflect safety and efficacy. Microbiologists look at the way anti-infective drugs act on viruses, bacteria, and other microbes.

In other words, when the FDA approves a drug for manufacture and sale, you can be certain that it has been examined and tested six ways till Sunday—and then some. And even after approval, the testing isn't over. Post-market surveys are done, and manufacturers are legally bound to report any and all adverse effects to the FDA.

After FDA approval, Phase IV trials are conducted. These are post-marketing studies that look at unexpected toxicity, gather data about new uses of the approved drug, refine dosing schedules, and seek additional information about long-term safety and efficacy.

You may want to refer back to this discussion of FDA approval when you read Chapter 11 on alternative medicine.

What FDA Approval Means

When the FDA approves a drug, it is saying that the company that developed it may manufacture and sell it for a specific indication, such as breast cancer. This does not mean that the drug is approved to treat lung cancer or prostate cancer or anything else. However, and this is a *big* however, physicians licensed to practice medicine are also licensed to prescribe whatever drugs they want to—for any reason. If this sounds like a paradox, it is. Off-label use of drugs—that is, prescribing them for conditions for which they have not been approved—carries two main advantages: it enables physicians to act on anecdotal evidence that a drug has shown benefit for a condition for which it has not yet been approved—without having to wait for approval—and it gives cancer patients who have not responded to standard chemotherapy the opportunity to try other drugs to which they may respond.

However, there also are two main disadvantages: incompetent and unknowledgeable physicians can use poor judgment when prescribing drugs, and health insurance companies and HMOs usually do not pay for off-label use.

Physicians Data Query

Physicians Data Query (PDQ) is a database maintained by the National Cancer Institute that contains summaries of about 1,500 ongoing clinical trials. The information it contains is free and available to the public (phone: (800) 345-3300; fax: (301) 402-5874). By contacting PDQ, you can find out the objectives and performance of each clinical trial; a discussion of biomedical, ethical, and other concerns for each trial; a list of all NCI-supported trials as well as other trials listed on a voluntary basis; names, addresses, phone numbers, and medical specialties of more than 20,000 oncologists; and about 2,500 organizations that provide cancer information and care. All information is updated at least monthly. The trials listed in PDQ are classified by research goals (prevention, cure, palliation, etc.); primary tumor type; treatment modality (chemotherapy, surgery, radiation); accrual (patient recruitment) status; study phase; and the drugs or biologicals being evaluated. Much of the same information is available at NCI's Web site: *www.nci.gov.*

Making Decisions

If a course or courses of chemotherapy does not cure your cancer (five years of complete remission is generally used as a benchmark for a cure), you may want to consider participation in a clinical trial. A new drug may do the trick, but even if it doesn't, it could improve the length and quality of your life by significantly relieving pain and other symptoms.

In addition, your oncologist might suggest a clinical trial because a drug or combination being tested is thought to be better than standard therapy. And if you have cancer of the prostate, colon, breast, or lung, or malignant melanoma (the top five cancers now being studied in the United States), your chances of finding an appropriate clinical trial are excellent.

Although about 80 percent of all oncologists participate in clinical research at some time during their careers—and more than 85 percent say that they view clinical trials as an essential way to improve patient care—only about 3 percent of all cancer patients participate in a clinical trial (between 40,000 and 45,000 people at any given time). In addition, only 1 to 2 percent of patients with the most common malignancies (breast, lung, or colon) are enrolled in a clinical trial. Most clinical trials are conducted at major cancer centers, but of the approximately 1 million Americans who are currently receiving cancer treatment, only a minority are treated at one of these centers.

There are major reasons for this divergence between physicians' stated interest and the obvious benefits of clinical trial participation and patient enrollment. For a variety of reasons, only about 20 percent of patients are eligible for any given trial, and of these, only half are approached by their oncologist—again for several reasons. Of the patients who apply for participation, less than half are actually enrolled.

Clinical trials usually have extremely stringent eligibility criteria, and critics have long urged relaxation of some of the requirements. This would create a much larger pool of potential participants, as well as more actual participants on whom to draw conclusions about safety and efficacy. On the other hand, if eligibility criteria were loosened beyond a certain point, the value of the data would be compromised.

Regardless of the advantages of clinical trials, there are certain things you ought to know before you sign up to participate in one. You want to know the purpose of the trial. The underlying purpose of all trials is to test one treatment against another, but each trial has its own particular agenda, and you should ask what that is. You also need to know what tests and treatments you will be required to undergo in addition to the drug or treatment under investigation: blood and other body fluid tests, physical examinations, imaging tests, and the like. Ask your oncologist what the standard treatment is for your cancer and how he or she evaluates the risks and benefits of standard treatment compared with the proposed investigational treatment.

There are other things you need to know.

How will participation in the study affect your day-to-day life? How often will you have to go to the cancer center for treatment and other tests and procedures? How far will you have to travel? Can you make it there and back in one day? Will you be able to drive, or will you always need to ask someone to accompany you? Is there a chance that you will have to be hospitalized?

How long will all this last, and how much and what type of follow-up will there be? How much will the ancillary care cost (the treatment itself is free), and will your insurance company pay for it? By the way, don't take the oncologist's or the assistant's word for this. Call your insurance company and find out. Get it in writing.

Cancer can be cured or well-treated in so many instances that it is now thought of as a chronic rather than an acute (and usually terminal) illness. Although the decision to undergo chemotherapy, with or without a clinical trial, is yours—and yours alone—if your physician suggests participating in a clinical trial, think positively about the opportunity you are being offered. A clinical trial may not be the most enjoyable experience you've ever had, but in the long run, you will be better off for having participated.

Chapter Seven

Side Effects

How to Cope with and Minimize
Treatment Side Effects

*P*ractically everyone knows someone who has had cancer, and you've probably heard that chemotherapy causes serious side effects—and that sometimes the treatment is worse than the disease. These perceptions have some truth and a great deal of falsity.

Cancer chemotherapy is *never* worse than having cancer. The side effects of treatment will go away when the treatment stops—and oftentimes even during treatment—whereas cancer, if left untreated, will eventually kill you. So if your physician recommends a course of chemotherapy, don't for one minute refuse *only because* you're afraid of the side effects.

Almost all side effects can be significantly minimized, and some can be eliminated entirely, and that's what you're going to learn in this chapter. Although many of the drugs do create some kind of side effects, they are not as bad as they were 10 years ago, and they're not nearly as bad as you've heard.

Regardless of how serious the side effects are and regardless of how they seem to be affecting your life, you should always report them to your oncologist. First, they may be indicative of something else. Second, he or she will want to follow their progress. And third, they can almost always be relieved by medication and/or other remedies.

Drugs and biologicals vary in the type and severity of the side effects they produce, and what's more, individual people vary tremendously in the way they react to drugs. Fear and anxiety usually make side effects worse, so if you're really scared of the drugs, tell your doctor, and he or she may give you anti-anxiety medication before each treatment begins. You also might want to use relaxation techniques or meditation while you are receiving the therapy. They have helped many people.

Learning about the drugs you will receive will provide powerful knowledge about why they do what they do—and why you react as you do. Knowing what's happening inside your body and what the drugs are doing to the healthy cells as well as the malignant ones can alleviate much fear and anxiety. In addition, knowledge is usually an anxiety reducer and an adjunct to a positive attitude. If you feel that the drugs are going to help, the side effects are more tolerable. In many respects, it's something like having surgery. You know that being cut open with a scalpel is going to cause a good deal of post-operative pain, but you also know two things: that whatever the surgeon is doing will be ultimately beneficial, and that the pain will be short-lived. In a week or so, except for the scar and some residual fatigue and soreness, you'll hardly remember that a surgeon was there.

No one experiences all the side effects that a given drug can produce, so don't panic when you read the lists that follow. Some lucky people have no side effects at all (but don't count on being one of those). Moreover, with very few exceptions, side effects (what physicians call *adverse events*) are predictable, which means they are manageable. That is, if a drug is known to make patients sick to their stomachs, an antiemetic can be given prior to or along with chemotherapy. If your hair is going to fall out, you know this beforehand so you can prepare for it in ways suggested here.

For more serious adverse events, especially those that affect blood and bone marrow, you will be followed closely and have your blood drawn at frequent intervals. Chemotherapy is *not* the equivalent of "take two aspirin and call me in the morning," so your body functions will be monitored more carefully than they ever have been before.

Why Side Effects Occur

It is a rule of thumb in medicine and pharmacology that any drug or other agent that is powerful enough to cause a positive effect is also powerful enough to cause a negative effect. This is particularly true of cancer chemotherapy, which consists of some of the most powerful drugs ever given to human beings. The reason why cancer drugs cause the effects they do is because they are designed to target cells that grow and divide quickly—cancer cells—as well as normal cells such as those in hair follicles and the gastrointestinal system.

Side effects run the gamut from a slight feeling of fatigue to lethal bone marrow depression. The vast majority will not kill you, but there are some events that you should report to your oncologist immediately:

➤ Fever of 100 degrees or more, especially with chills or shaking
➤ Allergic reaction such as hives or rash
➤ External bleeding, blood in the stool or urine, or black-and-blue marks that indicate internal bleeding
➤ Shortness of breath or chest pain that can signal cardiac problems
➤ Pain anywhere but especially at the injection site
➤ Severe diarrhea or constipation

Types of Side Effects

Immediate effects occur during or soon after treatment and disappear relatively quickly. The most common is nausea and vomiting, which we'll discuss again later. *Chronic effects* occur much later and last longer. The most common are fatigue, hair loss, sore mouth, depressed blood counts, and changes in bowel movements.

Biological Therapy

Although biological therapy was discussed in Chapter 4, a word or two here about side effects is appropriate. Almost all biological therapy consists of proteins and/or antibodies, both of which are destroyed by stomach acids. Thus, they must be given by injection, usually intravenous. The side effects vary with the type of biological agent and with the tissues they target, but there are a few general characteristics.

Tumor vaccines have few, if any, side effects, except possibly a low-grade fever or muscle aches, much like a slight case of the flu. *Cytokines* cause fever, fatigue, chills, skin rash, and possibly hypotension (low blood pressure). *Interferons* and *tumor necrosis factors* cause general malaise, again like the flu. *Interleukins*, especially IL-2, can cause severe life-threatening symptoms. The most worrisome is capillary leak syndrome, which is essentially what it sounds like: blood leaks out of capillaries, causing tissue swelling, hypotension, and kidney, cardiac, and respiratory problems. *Anti-tumor antibodies* can cause an allergic reaction of varying severity.

Hematologic Toxicity

Hematologic toxicity means side effects that affect the blood and its components. Most of the time, when *anemia, granulocytopenia, neutropenia,* or *thrombocytopenia* occur, they are the result of the toxic effects of the chemotherapy, but they also may be a result of the disease process itself.

When you begin a course of chemotherapy, your oncologist will keep a careful watch over your blood counts, so careful in fact that the constant testing of your blood will soon prove to be one of the most irritating things about chemotherapy, and all cancer patients learn to detest the sight of the "needle nurse."

Anemia and Fatigue

Anemia in cancer patients has a number of causes: blood loss, diminution of nutrients, infiltration of the bone marrow by tumor cells, bone marrow suppression caused by previous treatment, and the direct effects of cytotoxic drugs—the worst offenders being altretamine, cisplatin, cytarabine, paclitaxel, and topotecan.

One of the major consequences of anemia is severe fatigue. No one knows exactly what causes this most common side effect of chemotherapy (more than 90 percent of cancer patients experience it), but it probably has a great deal to do with thrombocytopenia, the diminution of red blood cells, which leads to anemia.

Other possible causes of fatigue include:

➤ Changes in the way the body processes nutrients and the fact that tumors compete for nutrients with normal cells—and tumor cells always win
➤ Other disease and treatment complications such as infection and fever

> The activities required of a cancer patient—the diagnostic tests, chemotherapy, and trips to the hospital and doctor's office resulting in changes in activity and rest patterns
> Fear, anxiety, stress, and worry about the future, which uses a lot of mental energy
> Pain
> Nausea and vomiting resulting in poor appetite
> Insomnia

Fatigue tends to be cyclical, in both its existence and severity; it is usually worst after a chemotherapy treatment. Many people say that the fatigue is the worst side effect of chemotherapy because it affects their entire lives and make them feel like a different person—one drained of energy and not a lot of fun to be around. It is pervasive and tends to drag on and on.

One of the major problems of fatigue is how it will affect your job. If you're so tired that you can't show up for work, you are forced to take a sick day. All employers provide a certain number of sick days, and when you use them up, that's it. Even short-term disability, which is a perk given by some employers, doesn't last forever. But even if you can make it to your desk or your place on the factory floor, you are not going to be as productive as usual, and eventually this will be noticed. And if you do work that requires constant alertness, you may even be a danger to yourself and your coworkers. Although it is not within the scope of this book to go into detail about your work situation, most cancer patients find that if they are candid about what's going on in their lives and if they have a frank discussion with the boss, they are better off than having to hide the illness and treatment—and have the boss think they are turning into a poor employee.

Prevention and Treatment
Serious fatigue really cannot be completely prevented, but you can do some things to minimize and cope with it:

> Eat as well as possible (pay special attention to proteins and carbohydrates) and drink lots of water.
> Do moderate exercise, such as walking or easy bicycle riding.

➤ Distract yourself with hobbies, reading, music, gardening, and the like.
➤ Treat insomnia—and ask your doctor for a prescription for a mild sedative or tranquilizer.
➤ Establish an activity and rest pattern that works well and learn to pace yourself.
➤ Take naps.
➤ Ask for help when you're too tired to do something—or know that you will be.
➤ Use relaxation techniques such as transcendental meditation, yoga, guided imagery, and the like.

Leukopenia, Neutropenia, and Infection

Leukopenia is a diminution of the total number of white blood cells. Neutropenia is a diminution of neutrophils, a type of granulocye (white blood cell). When the number of neutrophils falls below 1,500 cells/mm of blood, the risk of infection rises, and the seriousness of the infection is related to the degree and duration of the neutropenia.

Many chemotherapy drugs are *myelosuppressive*—that is, they depress the activity of the bone marrow, which produces the stem cells that mature into blood cells, and too few white blood cells can result in infection (see Chapter 3).

Since your oncologist knows which drugs are most likely to cause leukopenia, your white cell count will be followed very carefully; if it drops too low, the dose of the drug will have to be decreased or the drug stopped altogether until the counts rise again to safe levels. But before you reach this point, you might be given antibiotics or colony-stimulating factor to boost the white cell count.

Chemotherapy also affects the immune system, so the risk of infection increases. General causes of infection include:

➤ Breaching of the body's major defenses (skin and mucous membranes) by needle punctures as well as by the chemotherapeutic drugs themselves
➤ Reduction in the number of white blood cells
➤ Decrease in cellular immunity (T-lymphocytes) caused by some cancers (Hodgkin's disease and non-Hodgkin's lymphoma, for instance) and by chemotherapy

➤ Decrease in humoral immunity (B-lymphocytes) that produces antibodies that fight infection

Types of infection are:

1. Bacterial (strep throat and wound infections, for example), which derive from skin punctures, invasions of mucous membranes, and lack of resistance to organisms that normally live in the gastrointestinal tract
2. Viral (colds and the flu, for example), which are caused by cold sores and airborne microorganisms
3. Fungal (athlete's foot, for example), which are common when white blood cell counts are low

Before you begin a course of chemotherapy, you should learn the signs of present or impending infection, and when you have any of them, even one of them, *you must call the doctor immediately.* That phone call, which you should not be shy of making, can save your life. The signs of infection are:

➤ Temperature of 100 degrees or more
➤ Chills, with or without shaking
➤ Diarrhea for more than two days
➤ Burning with urination
➤ Cough, runny nose, chest pain, and other cold and flu symptoms
➤ Bleeding or discharge from vagina, rectum, bladder, or lungs
➤ Redness, pus, swelling, or heat in a wound

Prevention and Treatment
Three general things can be done by your physician to prevent or minimize infection during chemotherapy:

➤ Beef up the immune system by using hematopoietic growth factors, especially granulocyte colony-stimulating factor to reduce the severity and duration of neutropenia.
➤ Maintain the body's natural system of defense against infection by paying careful attention to protection of mechanical barriers such as skin and intestinal mucosa.

➤ Reduce exposure to environmental organisms by keeping patients out of the hospital as much as possible and maintaining good preventive techniques if people must be hospitalized.

Although your oncologist will decide if you need hematopoietic growth factors, antibiotics, or other drugs, there are a number of things you can do for yourself to prevent infection:

➤ Wash your hands with soap and water frequently. This is the single most important preventive measure. Take a bath or shower every day.

➤ Stay away from people who are sick. Even catching an ordinary cold can be devastating for someone with leukopenia or neutropenia. Don't be afraid of "insulting" people by postponing a lunch or dinner date until they're no longer contagious.

➤ If you must be hospitalized, make sure you get a private room. Most health insurance companies will pick up the extra cost if your doctor certifies that the room is medically necessary—and it is.

➤ Get a flu shot.

➤ Stay off airplanes or away from other enclosed spaces where air is recirculated. Viruses and bacteria abound in such places, and you have no means of escape.

➤ Avoid scratching or cutting yourself from gardening or other "dirty" activities such as cleaning the cat box or bird cage.

➤ Get sufficient rest or sleep.

➤ Avoid rectal contact during sex and make sure the vagina is well lubricated during sexual intercourse.

➤ Change your tampon frequently during menstruation.

➤ Maintain scrupulous cleanliness in the genital area (for both men and women).

➤ Try to eat what is called a low microbial diet by sticking to foods that tend to have a low bacteria count. Avoid the following: raw or rare meat; cold salads that contain meat, fish, or mayonnaise; processed lunch meats; pizza; raw vegetables or salads; fresh fruit; fried onion rings or French fries; raw or semi-cooked eggs; wine; dairy products that have passed their freshness date; nondairy whipped topping or coffee lightener; yogurt; cream-filled candy or pastries; nuts and candy bars; condiments that have been sitting out; ice cream; or water from an "iffy" municipal system.

Most infections can be successfully treated with antibiotics (which are effective only against bacteria) and anti-viral drugs, but if the causative agent (virus or bacterium) is particularly aggressive, your doctor may attempt to raise your white blood cell count during chemotherapy by giving colony-stimulating factor to "rescue" your white blood cells. By the way, white blood cells cannot be transfused.

In all likelihood you will be hospitalized while the infection is being treated because most antibiotics are given intravenously, and because a severe infection that arises from chemotherapy is life threatening. Your oncologist will want to keep careful watch over you—and probably will call in an infection specialist.

Thrombocytopenia

Thrombocytopenia is a low platelet count, a common and highly predictable side effect of many chemotherapeutic drugs such as carboplatin, dacarbazine, 5-FU, lomustine, mitomycin, streptozocin, thiotepa, and others.

The lower the platelet count, the greater the risk of bleeding, and in some instances the count may fall so low that the chemotherapy has to be stopped, or the dose lowered, until platelets return to near normal. It's also possible that you might require a blood transfusion.

When people think of serious bleeding, they usually imagine a cut that takes a long time to clot or a black-and-blue mark (which is capillary bleeding just under the skin) that takes a while to heal. But severe thrombocytopenia carries the risk of massive bleeding from places you can't see—the gastrointestinal tract, brain, and respiratory tract—all of which are life-threatening.

You should watch for symptoms that can signal thrombocytopenia: an increased tendency toward bruising; little red dots on your skin (called petechiae); bleeding gums; oozing of blood from any mucous membrane (mouth, vagina, nostrils, and such); blood in the stool, vomitus, or urine; excessive bleeding during menstruation (called hypermenorrhea); and bleeding during sexual intercourse.

Gastrointestinal Toxicity

Nausea and Vomiting

Nausea and vomiting result from a number of stimuli: the action of chemotherapeutic drugs on the rapidly growing cells that line the gastrointestinal system; triggering of the chemoreceptor zone in the brain, which can be stimulated by a number of different things, not just chemotherapy; intestinal obstruction; brain tumor; belief that the side effect will occur, called *anticipatory nausea and vomiting*; and severe anxiety.

The side effect known as nausea and vomiting actually has three components: nausea, retching, and actual vomiting. *Nausea* is an unpleasant sensation difficult to describe but familiar to and experienced by everyone at some time. It is generally characterized by a sense of uneasiness in the throat, stomach, and abdomen. Someone who is seriously nauseated is revolted by food—or even the thought of it (oddly, mild nausea can be eased by eating a small amount of something bland and light)—and feels unable to carry on with normal activities.

Retching is a rhythmic spasmodic movement of the chest, diaphragm, and stomach muscles that precedes vomiting but doesn't always result in vomiting. If vomiting does not ensue, retching is often referred to as the "dry heaves." *Vomiting* is the forceful expulsion through the mouth or nose of the contents of the stomach or upper small intestine.

Chemotherapy generally produces three patterns of nausea and vomiting: acute, delayed, and anticipatory. Acute nausea and vomiting occur within the first 24 hours of treatment and are almost always related to the propensity of the drug to cause sickness, the route of administration, the dose, and often the time of day the drug is given. Delayed nausea occurs more than a day after treatment, lasts from one to seven days, with a peak on Day 3. Even when *antiemetics* effectively prevent acute nausea, delayed sickness is not uncommon. Antiemetics work well for delayed vomiting but not so well for nausea, which can become problematic because it can adversely affect nutrition and it has a pervasive negative effect on well-being.

Anticipatory nausea and vomiting (ANV) is a phenomenon uniquely associated with chemotherapy. It is defined as experiencing one or both of these symptoms *before* receiving a dose of chemotherapy. It is a conditioned response to the prior experience of getting sick over the drugs, and it can be very severe. Some people experience nausea when they even think about chemotherapy, and it's not uncommon to throw up on the way to the hospital or clinic. Some people feel sick on exposure to certain odors associated with the chemotherapy experience: rubbing alcohol, the plastic tubing—even a certain perfume worn by a chemotherapy nurse. Anticipatory nausea is *not* all in your head; it is a very powerful and frustrating experience. If you are reading this before you begin treatment, you may find it difficult to believe that just driving past the treatment center (or bumping into a chemotherapy nurse on the street—or thinking about chemotherapy) can induce powerful nausea. But it's true.

The best way to deal with anticipatory nausea is to prevent it. First, don't do any of the things that you know will trigger nausea. Don't accompany a friend to his or her doctor's office if you know you're going to feel sick. Stay away from hospital programs on television if they make you clap your hand over your mouth and bolt for the bathroom. Don't drive anywhere near the hospital. And if a "chemotherapy thought" pops into your head (it's hard to stop thinking about it because it's such a central part of your life right now), immediately use relaxation techniques to stop the nausea. Breathe deeply with your mouth open, relax your muscles, force yourself to think about something pleasant and calming, and visualize yourself feeling fine.

Since ANV can strike at any time, and since you won't always be successful at controlling it, carry a "barf bag" with you at all times. The kind the airlines put in the seat pocket is best (call an airline and ask to purchase a dozen or so or ask a frequent flyer friend to bring you a few from his or her next flight), but a strong plastic bag will work.

Drugs most likely to cause nausea and vomiting are cisplatin, cyclophosphamide, daunorubicin, doxorubicin, dacarbazine, mechlorethamine, and streptozocin. Drugs with a moderate likelihood of making you sick are carboplatin, cytarabine, carmustine, methyl-CCNU, etoposide, ifosfamide, methotrexate, mitomycin, lomustine, and procarbazine. No one seems to know why some drugs are more likely than others to cause nausea and vomiting—and why some people are more susceptible to queasiness than others.

When the chemotherapy treatment begins, you will start to feel sick either after a few minutes or after a few hours. Some people can

make it home before they begin retching, and some can't make it out
the door of the treatment room.

Even though you feel as though you might die of persistent
retching (some people never actually vomit), no one ever does, and
although it feels horrible, it is not one of the most serious side effects
of chemotherapy. But by the same token, if nausea and vomiting are
left unchecked and untreated, they can cause a number of problems.
Patients can become so "freaked out" by it that they stop treatment.
In addition, it can result in dehydration, serious weight loss, severe
fatigue, and electrolyte imbalance serious enough to cause respiratory and cardiac problems, lethargy, and convulsions. If retching is
strong and protracted, your back and ribs can hurt, and there have
even been cases of rib fracture.

Prevention and Treatment

Now, before you back off and say that you don't want any part
of chemotherapy—or before you run off to the bathroom to throw
up out of anxiety-induced anticipation—know that there are excellent drugs now given routinely to prevent, or at least minimize,
nausea and vomiting. They are called antiemetics (the medical term
for vomiting is *emesis*) and include the following drugs:

> ➤ Prochlorperazine (Compazine) is administered orally, rectally
>   in a suppository, intramuscularly, or intravenously. It can
>   cause drowsiness, sometimes to the extent that you shouldn't
>   drive home from the hospital or doctor's office, and it is not
>   always effective. Perphenazine (Trilafon) and thiethylperazine
>   (Torecan) belong to the same class of drug (phenothiazine) as
>   Compazine and have similar side effects. Most phenothiazines
>   work well in some patients but not others.
>
> ➤ Lorazepam (Ativan) and diazepam (Valium) are tranquilizers
>   that, strictly speaking, are not antiemetics. They make you
>   sleepy, relaxed, and drowsy and depress certain parts of your
>   brain so you "forget" to be nauseated. They are given orally,
>   intramuscularly, or intravenously, and again you shouldn't
>   drive home until their effects have worn off.
>
> ➤ Haloperidol (Haldol) and droperidol (Innovar) belong to a
>   class called butyrophenomes. They are administered orally

(Haldol), intramuscularly, or intravenously and are often used for patients who do not respond well to phenothiazines.

➤ Ondansetron (Zofran) is a fairly new drug and works by suppressing serotonin, a neurochemical that is often released by chemotherapy. Zofran is extremely effective and is often given intravenously right before chemotherapy and again afterward—or in a big dose an hour before treatment. Its effects last for 24 hours, and if nausea continues beyond that time, you can take it in pill form at home. One big advantage of Zofran is that it does not cause drowsiness, but it can make you constipated, so drink lots of water, take a stool softener, and use a laxative if you need one after a day or two.

➤ Granisetron (Kytril) is similar to Zofran.

➤ Metoclopramide (Reglan) is a dopamine (another neurochemical) antagonist. When given in high doses intravenously, it is very effective against the nausea and vomiting of cisplatin, one of the most notorious chemotherapeutic agents when it comes to nausea.

➤ Corticosteroids such as dexamethasone (Decadron) and methylprednisalone work well when given in high doses.

➤ Marijuana, although illegal when bought on the street, and hampered by miles of red tape when prescribed by an oncologist, is a highly effective antiemetic. It also lowers anxiety and creates a sense of well being. Side effects may include dizziness, paranoia, inability to concentrate, and accelerated heart rate. Because it is an illegal substance, you may want to think twice about using it, but if you have ever used it for recreational purposes, you will be familiar with its effects and will thus have an idea of how it may help during chemotherapy.

Antiemetics are given prior to the start of chemotherapy, usually by several hours, and preferably in a rectal suppository because they seem better tolerated that way. It's easy to do: take off the foil, lubricate the tip, and slip it into your rectum. Antiemetic medication should be continued for a day or two after each treatment.

Although antiemetic medications can be a godsend, there are things you can do for yourself to minimize the amount of nausea and vomiting you experience. Ask for a private room when you are actually receiving treatment. Although it's good to talk to other cancer patients in the waiting room and to share experiences and learn things, it's not a good idea to watch other people throw up. Neither do you want other people watching and listening to you. Use relaxation techniques prior to chemotherapy, including progressive muscle relaxation. Avoid offensive odors and sights. For instance, don't drive by the paper manufacturing plant, don't have your living room redone, and don't watch gory or grizzly movies while you are on chemotherapy. Try visualization techniques to see yourself as a cancer patient who doesn't have to vomit.

While you're feeling nauseated, you're not going to feel much like eating (and some people have a low-level "background" sort of nausea the entire time they're on chemotherapy), but of course you have to eat. Here are some techniques you can try to control the queasiness:

- ➤ Do what pregnant women do when they have morning sickness: eat some dry crackers, dry toast, or dry cereal before getting out of bed. Keep these things in your night table so you can eat before your feet hit the floor.
- ➤ Drink plenty of fluids so you don't become dehydrated. It's easier to tolerate clear liquids (water, ginger ale, apple juice, bouillon, and gelatin) than it is dairy products or soups such as chowders, minestrone, chunky chicken or meat soup, and the like. Many people find that carbonated beverages stay down better than still ones, but others say that the gas that induces burping might induce vomiting as well. Experiment and find out what works best for you.
- ➤ Anything that's overly sweet, overly spicy, or very highly flavored is hard to keep down when you're nauseated.
- ➤ Foods eaten cool or at room temperature tend not to be as strongly flavored as hot foods and are thus less likely to induce nausea.
- ➤ Don't stuff yourself. Eat when you're hungry, and eat small amounts of food at one time. You are not obligated to eat "three squares" a day.
- ➤ Ask other family members to do the cooking and stay out of the kitchen so the smell of food doesn't nauseate you. If you

live alone, you may be best off living on takeout food while you're on chemotherapy.

➤ While you're in the throes of serious nausea and vomiting, it's hard to think about anything else. But when the acute sickness passes and you're left with mild nausea, try to think about and do other things. Read, go to the movies, take a walk, weed the garden, visit friends.

➤ Mild exercise can ease nausea, but don't do anything strenuous right after eating because it may increase nausea and even induce vomiting.

➤ Try acupuncture or acupressure (see Chapter 11). It may or may not help you, but it's worth a try.

➤ Try deep breathing with your mouth slightly open, preferably outdoors in the fresh air, when you're feeling nauseated.

Anorexia

Anorexia means loss of appetite and is one of the most common side effects of chemotherapy. It is not the same as the eating disorder called anorexia nervosa. It is caused by *mucositis* (inflammation and soreness of the inside of the mouth); difficulty swallowing; stress and anxiety; other side effects of the chemotherapy, such as diarrhea; the disease itself, such as tumors in the bowel or esophagus; and a change in taste or smell of certain foods caused by some drugs. Almost everyone experiences appetite loss at one time or another during chemotherapy and the course of their disease, and weight loss of up to 15 or 20 pounds is common. Some people lose so much weight that they suffer from a condition called *cachexia*, which is a general wasting away of the body's tissues, especially muscle mass. It's fairly easy to recognize; sufferers look like pictures of famine victims. However, cachexia is usually confined to people dying of cancer (and other terminal diseases), so don't worry too much about it.

But you should worry about losing too much weight. Even if you were overweight to begin with, chemotherapy is *not* the way to go on a diet. Significant weight loss will weaken you and make it more difficult to tolerate the rigors of chemotherapy, and if you lose too much weight, you may not be able to tolerate the chemotherapy and will need to have the dose reduced or the drug stopped completely until you regain some weight.

Prevention and Treatment

Use all the techniques listed in the previous section on combating nausea and vomiting. In addition:

➤ Eat only what you like and what you know will go down easily and stay down.

➤ Learn what foods don't agree with you and avoid them.

➤ Don't skip meals. Lots of times you won't feel like eating, but do it anyway. If you really don't want to eat, think of a snack or small meal as "medicine."

➤ When you do eat, pack the most amount of nutrients and calories into the smallest amount of food. That way, you won't have to stuff yourself in order to be well nourished. But don't be unreasonably strict with yourself. If you hate cottage cheese, don't eat it. Have a wedge of brie or cheddar instead. If fish is too smelly, eat a lamb chop. If you love bacon, go ahead and enjoy it. This is not the time to worry about fat and cholesterol.

➤ Eat in a pleasant environment. If you're dining out, choose a nice restaurant (and don't sit near the kitchen door), eat outdoors if the weather is nice—and avoid greasy, smelly fast food joints. When you're home, set the table with nice dishes and linens, put a flower or two on the table, light a candle, listen to soothing music.

➤ Ask your doctor for an appetite stimulant such as prednisone, Megace (a form of progesterone), and Marinol.

➤ Learn what depresses your appetite and try to correct or prevent those factors. For example, if you are in pain, ask your doctor for medication. If you're stressed out, try relaxation techniques. If you're constipated, use a laxative or take an enema.

➤ Keep your mouth clean and fresh. Brush your teeth often, use mouthwash, and drink lots of water.

➤ Take a short walk before lunch or dinner. Mild exercise is a good appetite stimulant.

➤ It might be helpful to consult a *nutritionist*. The hospital will have one, or you can hire an independent consultant. Nutritionists (also called *dietitians*) have much experience with cancer patients, and they can devise food plans that provide the most nutrients with maximum palatability.

➤ If all else fails, drink nutrition supplements—the kind that nursing home patients use. These are high-calorie, high-protein drinks (or puddings) that come in a variety of flavors. They don't taste bad and are even better when they're cold and perked up with a scoop of ice cream or whizzed in a blender or food processor with fruit or flavor extracts. You can also freeze the supplement and eat it like a Popsicle. But because the supplements have no bulk, beware of constipation.

Stomatitis

Chemotherapeutic drugs have some of the same irritating effects on the lining of the mouth as on the gastrointestinal tract because the tissue is the same. This can lead to a condition called *stomatitis* (also called *mucositis*), an inflammation of the mouth and throat, which can cause ulcerations if it becomes severe. It goes away shortly after treatment is discontinued (although the healing process will take longer if your nutrition is compromised), but while it is going on, it is highly unpleasant and painful. You won't feel much like eating because some foods hurt your mouth. But if you don't eat, you'll lose weight and run the risk of becoming dehydrated. This is to be avoided.

You also might find that the taste of food changes, and it's usually not a change for the better. Fortunately, this is not a permanent state of affairs.

Prevention and Treatment

There's not a lot you can do to prevent having a sore mouth (and throat too sometimes), but you can minimize the symptoms. Use good oral hygiene with a soft toothbrush. (Try a foam swab or commercial tooth towelettes if a brush is too irritating.) Floss after every meal because food stuck between teeth can be a major irritant and can lead to cavities and gum problems. Avoid major dental (including periodontal) work during chemotherapy, but do have it done before you embark on a course of chemotherapy. Also, have your teeth cleaned before you begin chemotherapy—and tell your dentist that you have cancer and what drugs you will be taking. He or she may have suggestions about treating sore mouth. If you wear dentures or have a removable bridge, brush them two or three times a day (they provide excellent places for harboring bacteria) and put them in water until you have thoroughly cleaned the inside of your mouth, preferably with commercial mouthwash that contains an antibacterial or antiseptic. If you find that your mouthwash stings or burns, ask you dentist for a suggestion for a milder one.

Keep your mouth moist with liquids, hard candies, and the like. Use lip balm or lipstick, and treat all mouth infections (herpes, monilia, etc.) immediately.

Maintain adequate nutrition (perhaps with the help of a nutritionist), avoid foods that hurt your mouth, *don't smoke*, *avoid alcohol*, and ask your doctor for medication, such as a topical spray of lidocaine, to treat particularly severe mouth pain.

If you have mouth ulcers, buy a bottle of milk of magnesia. Several times a day, swish some around your mouth and spit it out—but don't rinse. It may not taste too wonderful, but it's very soothing.

Diarrhea

Diarrhea, which occurs in about 75 percent of all chemotherapy patients at one time or another, is almost always temporary, but it is extremely annoying while it's happening. It's no fun to feel as though you can't step more than two feet from a bathroom. Chemotherapeutic drugs, as well as some antibiotics, cause diarrhea. The intestines react to the irritation of the drugs by speeding up in an effort to pass the irritant through the system as quickly as possible.

The biggest culprits for causing diarrhea include aminocamptothecin, cytabarine, dactinomycin, 5-FU, hydroxyurea, irinotecan, methotrexate, mitotane, and topotecan. As with all other adverse events, the dose, schedule, and route of administration affect the incidence and severity of diarrhea.

Symptoms include loose stools several times a day, a feeling of urgency, excess amounts of gas (called *flatulence*), abdominal cramps, and soreness around the anus (treat yourself to the softest toilet paper you can buy).

If diarrhea is allowed to continue unchecked, it can cause dehydration, weakness, weight loss, and even malnutrition, and chemical imbalances resulting from diminished absorption of nutrients.

Prevention and Treatment

To prevent or minimize occasional diarrhea, avoid greasy and spicy foods, caffeine, citrus fruits, and foods that are high in bulk and fiber such as whole grain breads and cereals, popcorn, nuts, and raw vegetables.

If diarrhea continues for more than a couple of days, call the doctor. But in the meantime, eat a diet that allows the bowels to rest, a diet that consists of mostly liquids and very soothing foods such as eggs, custard, soft cheeses, cooked cereal, mild meats (chicken and lamb, for instance), bananas, applesauce, potatoes, and noodles (you might consult a professional nutritionist). Drink plenty of mild liquids at room temperature (to replenish the fluids lost through loose stools), avoid very hot or very cold foods and liquids, "defizz" carbonated beverages, and take an anti-diarrhea medication such as Lomotil or Kaopectate.

Concentrate on foods that are high in protein and calories and that are high in potassium (loss of fluids tends to deplete potassium). In addition, there are foods you ought to avoid:

- ➤ Whole grains and high-fiber foods
- ➤ Most everything recommended as a treatment for constipation
- ➤ Strong, spicy foods such as hot peppers, horseradish, chili, and the like
- ➤ Caffeine
- ➤ Milk
- ➤ Chocolate

Since you know your body better than anyone else, give up foods that have tended to give you diarrhea in the past.

As with all other digestive upsets, small, frequent meals are better than three large ones in controlling diarrhea. And you need to be careful about getting sufficient nutrients, especially protein and potassium.

If you have abdominal cramps, use a hot water bottle or heating pad (or lie down and invite your cat to sit on your belly), or take a warm bath. Diarrhea can be extremely exhausting, so be sure to get sufficient sleep and rest. If your anus becomes irritated as a result of frequent trips to the bathroom, use a topical anesthetic like Tucks or benzocaine.

Constipation

Constipation is caused by dietary changes, especially too little fiber or high-bulk foods; chemotherapeutic drugs; opiates and other drugs; stress; and lack of exercise.

Because you have not moved your bowels for a day or two does not mean you are constipated. Not everyone has a bowel movement (BM) every day; nor is it necessarily normal to be on a daily routine. You know you're constipated when you have skipped a BM for longer than is *usual for you*, when your stool is hard or darker than usual (which means that it has been sitting in your large intestine losing water content), and when you have to strain to have a bowel movement. Severe constipation can cause abdominal distention and cramping, decreased appetite, and fecal impaction. The latter is a hard mass of feces stuck in the rectum or lower colon which no amount of pushing and straining will dislodge. It is no fun at all and has to be removed manually.

You should report constipation to your oncologist because it is a side effect of several chemotherapeutic agents. It usually does not appear until after a few drug cycles and can be accompanied by tingling or numbness in fingers and toes. This may signal the beginning of neurotoxicity and can be potentially serious.

Prevention and Treatment

Constipation is fairly easy to prevent and treat, but you should take care of it at the outset because you definitely do not want it to get worse. These are things you can do:

➤ Eat a high-fiber, high-bulk diet with lots of fresh fruit and vegetables. You don't have to eat all vegetables raw, but cook them only until they're done but still crisp. Nuts, cereal, and popcorn also are good.

➤ Find ways to add extra bran to your diet. Eat bran cereals and muffins, and add bran to recipes when you make meatloaf, pancakes, cookies, and other baked goods. When you get tired of bran cereal, sprinkle bran on other types of cereal.

➤ Drink at least eight glasses of water a day. This helps keep your stool soft.

➤ Drinking hot liquids (but not tea or coffee because they are mild diuretics and tend to deplete the body of water) may stimulate bowel activity.

➤ Avoid foods that you have found to be constipating in the past, such as white bread, starchy desserts, chocolate, and the like.

➤ If you can manage it, eat a large breakfast with a hot beverage such as decaffeinated coffee or herbal tea.

➤ Exercise as much as you can.

➤ Use a stool softener such as Colace every night before you go to bed. Or you can take the Colace in the morning and then sit in a warm bath before you go to bed. This will relax your anal sphincter, and you may have a bowel movement when you get out of the tub.

➤ Take a mild laxative if necessary, or a strong laxative if that doesn't work, in order to avoid fecal impaction. You can also try a suppository (start with glycerin before going on to something stronger like Dulcolox) or an enema.

➤ When you're in the bathroom, take your time. Don't feel rushed, and don't let other members of the family try to hurry you.

Dermatological Toxicity

Alopecia

Alopecia (hair loss) is one of the most emotionally devastating side effects. It occurs because the cells in hair follicles grow and divide particularly rapidly and thus are highly vulnerable to some, but not all, chemotherapeutic drugs. Cyclophosphamide, adriamycin, aminocamptothecin, doxorubicin, dactinomycin, irinotecan, paclitaxel, topotecan, and vincristine are among the worst offenders. About 85 percent of all chemotherapy patients lose all or some of their hair, and again, hair loss depends very much on the drug or combination, dosage, and route of administration.

If your hair is going to fall out, there is nothing you can do to prevent it, but try to remember one thing as you weep over the clumps of hair that cling to your comb and brush: *It will grow back.* You will not be bald for the rest of your life. And you may not lose all your hair; rather, it may become thin and patchy, which many people, especially women, think is worse than total baldness.

And it's not just the hair on the top of your head that is affected. Men will lose their mustaches and beards, and both sexes will lose eyebrows and eyelashes, which many women say bothers them more than losing head hair. Body hair also is affected, although sometimes it doesn't fall out completely.

Alopecia is one of the most medically insignificant side effects of chemotherapy because it in no way endangers your health, but people hate it because it *shows* so glaringly. Totally bald men are not particularly noticeable in American society, especially during the fashion trend of deliberately shaved heads, but women stand out like sore thumbs—or cancer patients. Hair loss thus adds insult to injury, and can throw some people into a depression as severe as that which they experienced when they first found out they had cancer.

On the other hand, some patients react almost casually to alopecia—particularly in view of everything else they have to endure as a cancer patient. Some see it as visual proof that the drugs are working, some see wigs as an opportunity to try life with a different hair color, and others simply accept it as part of the treatment.

Hair loss usually begins during the first cycle of treatment, and starts to grow back three to six months later. Sometimes the new growth of hair is slightly changed in texture and/or color.

Preparation and Treatment

Before you begin chemotherapy, ask your doctor if the drugs will cause hair loss, and if so, prepare yourself emotionally and physically. First, get your hair cut short (and men should shave off their beards and mustaches) before you begin treatment so the loss won't be as devastating or noticeable to others. Second, go to a wig store and try some on before you need one. If you want to, experiment with different hair colors, or variations on your own color, and styles. Do tell the salesperson that you are about to embark on a course of chemotherapy; most are very sympathetic and have experience working with cancer patients. You might even ask the staff in your oncologist's office to recommend a wig maker; they probably know every one in town. And by the way, wigs are usually covered by health insurance for cancer patients, so get a good one.

If you think you will want to wear a wig, buy one *before* your hair falls out. Even if you end up accepting alopecia relatively philosophically, everyone is shocked to varying points of devastation when it first happens. Your appearance is totally changed by baldness, and wearing a wig will soften the shock somewhat.

If you choose not to wear a wig, buy a few hair coverings (scarves, turbans, hats, etc.) before treatment begins; you can always get more later. If you go outdoors without your wig or scarf, don't forget to put sunscreen on your head. Not only is sunscreen a good idea in general, but your newly bald scalp will be especially vulnerable to ultraviolet rays. Wear a hat in cold weather even if you usually don't, because a large percentage of body heat is lost through the head, and you will no longer have hair to act as insulation.

When treatment begins, use a mild shampoo, don't rub hard, and don't brush or comb vigorously. Don't use a hair dryer, hot rollers, or a curling iron; they speed up hair loss. Putting a tight band around your scalp during chemotherapy sometimes minimizes hair loss, but don't be disappointed if this doesn't work—or if you just don't want to bother with it.

You may have heard about the technique of scalp cooling (*hypothermia*) during chemotherapy administration as a way to prevent or minimize hair loss. Don't try it. Not only does it almost never work, it can be dangerous for people with scalp metastases of solid tumors or for people at high risk for central nervous system dissemination, and for people with cutaneous T-cell lymphoma. Even though scalp metastasis is very rare, the FDA banned commercial sale of scalp-cooling devices, and you will be hard-pressed to find a hospital or clinic that knows how to use this preventive measure.

Other Dermatological Side Effects

Almost all skin changes are self-limiting; that is, they last only as long as you are receiving chemotherapy. Some can be annoying and severe while they are going on, but none is life-threatening, and almost none is dose-limiting. Some common skin reactions are:

➤ Fingernails can become darkened, brittle, and grow more slowly.
➤ Skin and mucous membranes also may get darker (called hyperpigmentation), either in patches or all over.

➤ Other skin changes include dryness, itchiness, or flakiness, which makes it more susceptible to bacterial and fungal infections.

➤ Tender red patches may appear on the soles of the feet and palms of the hands. This is called palmar-plantar erythrodysesthesia syndrome, more commonly referred to as hand-foot syndrome, and it can be quite painful. It is most commonly associated with cytabarine, doxorubicin, and 5-FU. If you get severe hand-foot syndrome, your doctor will give you a prescription for pain relief (topical and systemic). You also should keep your feet elevated and do your best to prevent the sores from becoming infected.

Renal Toxicity

Chemotherapy drugs most likely to cause *renal toxicity* (kidney problems) are L-aspariginase, carboplatin, cisplatin, hydroxyurea, ifosfamide, methotrexate, mitomycin, pentostatin, plicamycin, streptozocin, and suramin. Complicating factors are age, nutritional status, prior or concurrent use of other nephrotoxic drugs (those that have a deleterious effect on the kidneys), and pre-existing kidney disease.

One of the major problems of impaired kidney function, in addition to the damage to the kidneys themselves, is the effect it has on other organ systems, such as the nervous and reproductive systems.

Before you begin a course of chemotherapy, you may be asked to collect your urine for 24 hours to determine levels of blood urea nitrogen and creatinine, two important measures of kidney function. If there is a problem, your oncologist may choose another drug, or give you the original drug and test your urine very frequently. In any event, one of the most important things you can do to prevent or minimize renal toxicity is to drink *lots* of water—at least eight glasses a day.

Bladder Toxicity

Cyclophosphamide and ifosfamide are associated with hemorrhagic cystitis (inflammation of the bladder accompanied by bleeding), as well as increased risk of bladder carcinoma, especially when given in high doses.

Bladder toxicity is caused when metabolites (chemical end products) of these and other drugs come into contact with the delicate bladder wall lining. The result is erythema (redness), inflammation, ulceration, necrosis (death of tissue), tiny oozing hemorrhages, and a reduced bladder capacity. These things will manifest themselves as a series of symptoms: blood in the urine (hematuria), which you may or may not be able to see; pain on urination; and increased frequency and urgency of urination.

Bladder toxicity is treated by significantly increasing fluid intake (if you don't drink enough water, you'll be put in the hospital and given intravenous fluids), sometimes irrigating the bladder through an indwelling catheter to reduce the concentration of the irritating substances, and sometimes fulguration (destruction of necrotic tissues by sparking them with electricity).

Pulmonary Toxicity

Damage to lung tissue as a result of chemotherapy is of three types: *pneumonitis* or *fibrosis*, *hypersensitivity pneumonitis* and *noncardiogenic pulmonary edema*. Pneumonitis is inflammation of the lung tissue; fibrosis is an abnormality of a certain type of tissue in the lung; pulmonary edema is fluid in the lungs (noncardiogenic means that it does not involve the heart).

What all this means to you is that if you develop pulmonary complications, you will cough, have some difficulty breathing, and may have chest pain and shortness of breath.

When you develop any of these symptoms, you'll have a chest x-ray and perhaps a series of tests to measure pulmonary function. If there is serious lung damage, either the dose of the drug will be reduced or you will be switched to another regimen. You may be put on corticosteroid drugs for a while, and will recover quickly. The important thing is to report the symptoms to your oncologist when they first appear, because pulmonary toxicity can be quickly and easily treated when it is still in the early stage. But the more severe it is and the longer it goes on, the more likely you are to have permanent lung damage.

Cardiac Toxicity

The most common and most serious cardiac side effects are *congestive heart failure* (due to an excess of fluid) and *cardiomyopathy* (damage to the heart muscle itself) associated with doxorubicin and other anthracycline drugs. Other cardiac effects such as *ischemia* (insufficient oxygen to the heart muscle), *pericarditis* (inflammation of the sac surrounding the heart), *arrhythmias* (dysfunction in the rhythm of the heartbeat), and *angina* (chest pain) occur less often.

Cardiac toxicity, especially from doxorubicin, can be acute (occurring within hours of administration), chronic (occurring weeks, months, or even a year after therapy), or late onset (occurring more than a year after treatment).

Acute cardiac toxicity tends to be transient and not dose-related, and it usually does not portend future cardiac problems. Chronic and late onset toxicity, on the other hand, are dose-related (especially as regards total cumulative dose) and can result in permanent heart damage.

Early detection is the best way to manage cardiac toxicity, so if you are taking doxorubicin or other related drugs, you will have frequent electrocardiograms and perhaps echocardiograms and angiocardiograms, all of which are noninvasive (no one sticks needles or instruments into you) and painless. You also should have long-term cardiac follow-up care after you have completed the chemotherapy because, although the incidence of cardiac failure is low, it does exist. If you do experience cardiac problems as a result of doxorubicin therapy, you will be given conventional treatment for heart failure.

Neurological Toxicity

Chemotherapy can affect the nervous system in a wide variety of ways and in a wide range of severity. That's the bad news; the good news is that serious *neurological toxicity* is relatively rare and almost always progresses from mild warning signs to more severe symptoms so that a particular drug regimen can be stopped or the dose modified before a patient gets into real neurological trouble.

Common dysfunctions include *encephalopathy* (brain dysfunction), *peripheral neuropathy* (dysfunction of the nerves in the arms, legs, hands, and feet), *cerebellar syndrome* (dysfunction of the cerebellum, which controls voluntary muscles), *autonomic neuropathy* (disease of the autonomic nervous system, which controls involuntary functions such as digestion and respiration), and *cranial nerve toxicity* (causing vision and hearing problems). As with other types of toxicities, those affecting the neurological systems are a function of the drug or combination, dose, route of administration, use of other neurotoxic drugs in conjunction with cancer chemotherapy, radiotherapy of the brain or spinal cord (together known as the central nervous system), as well as previous neurological problems.

The list of symptoms is long, but most are mild, and many disappear by themselves even before chemotherapy is finished. You may experience one or more of the following: difficulty concentrating; memory problems; sluggish thinking; impaired ability to coordinate movements; impaired vision, hearing, or other senses; trouble doing mathematical calculations; depression; apathy; confusion; and headache. Regardless of how innocuous you think your symptoms are, you *must* report them to your oncologist so he or she can evaluate them and make a decision about continuing therapy.

Gonadal Toxicity

The effects of chemotherapy and hormone therapy on the *gonads* (ovaries and testes) and on reproductive function vary. Alkylating agents are the most seriously toxic and can result in testicular atrophy and ovarian failure. Young adults and children suffer the most adverse consequences of gonadal toxicity not only because they are or soon will be of childbearing age, but because their gonadal cells are at their most active and are thus highly vulnerable to cytotoxic drugs.

The drugs most likely to cause gonadal toxicity are mustargen, oncovin, procarbazine, and prednisone.

In women, as age increases, there is decreasing likelihood of ovarian dysfunction; when it occurs, it is usually manifested as amenorrhea (absence of menstruation) and failure to ovulate. In men, the nature of the malignancy seems to be as important a factor as the chemotherapeutic drug in terms of gonadal dysfunction, which is manifested as impotence, low sperm counts, or absence of sperm. Other symptoms in both sexes include loss of libido, hot flashes, mood changes, vaginal discharge in women, and gynecomastia (enlargement of the breasts) in men.

Sexual Activity

Since sexual arousal and the ability to engage in sexual activity is a function of combined physical and emotional factors, when your physical and emotional being are not in tiptop shape, your sex life is going to suffer from the effects of both the chemotherapy and the cancer itself. The lack of desire for sex almost always returns either when chemotherapy side effects subside or when the course of treatment is finished, but before that time, your sex life (or lack of it) can be a frustrating experience—for you and for your partner.

Men

A number of chemotherapeutic drugs such as cisplatin and vincristine can affect the nerves that cause erectile function, and temporary impotence may result. However, most men taking most drugs are able to have perfectly normal erections. Still, because of other side effects, sexual desire may not be what it was before the cancer. After all, the thought of having intercourse is not too appealing when you're nauseated or in the throes of diarrhea.

Hormone therapy for prostate cancer or surgery for testicular cancer can have a negative effect on the ability to achieve and maintain an erection. Older men have more serious problems in this area than do younger ones.

Some drugs—vincristine, again—can damage the nerves that control emission of semen, so although there is orgasm with all its attendant pleasure, there is no ejaculation.

Some chemotherapeutic drugs and some used to control nausea cause decreased production of testosterone, a male hormone that plays a significant role in sexual desire. Therefore, although you *can* have sex, you may not feel much like it until after you have stopped taking those drugs.

Women

Women suffer from the same loss of desire for sex that men do (and not feeling or looking your best can have an enormous effect on sexual desire even if strictly physical side effects do not). But desire returns eventually.

Hormone therapy such as tamoxifen for breast cancer can cause menopausal symptoms such as hot flashes, vaginal dryness, and diminished libido. Androgens, also used sometimes to treat breast cancer, can increase sexual desire, but given in high doses, it causes masculization symptoms: deepened voice, acne, and increased facial hair. Although these changes can be very upsetting, they almost always disappear when the therapy is stopped.

Much more problematic for women who have not had all the children they want is the possibility of premature menopause: permanent destruction of ovarian function as a direct result of chemotherapy, especially combination therapy. Less drastic but almost as problematic is when ovarian and menstrual function recover after chemotherapy but menopause occurs much earlier than normal—another form of premature menopause.

Some experimentation has been done in removing and freezing ova prior to the initiation of chemotherapy, but it should be emphasized that this research is in its very earliest investigational phase and ultimately may not be workable. Even if it does work, it is a surgical procedure, and most women don't want to face surgery in addition to chemotherapy.

Other sexual side effects include: vaginal dryness that makes intercourse uncomfortable or painful (various estrogen creams and other lubricants can help with this); hot flashes; partial loss of vaginal elasticity; and an increased vulnerability to yeast infections, genital herpes, and warts.

Chapter Eight

Radiation and Surgery

Two Other Ways to Treat Cancer Often Used in Conjunction with Chemotherapy

Radiation

Radiation therapy (also called *radiotherapy*) is the process of sending radioactive atoms into the body to accomplish two major things: to visualize internal body parts (x-rays and various imaging techniques such as CAT scans and barium studies); and to kill cancer cells by damaging their DNA. Radiation is used frequently as a treatment for cancer, often in combination with surgery and/or chemotherapy.

Atoms, as you may remember from high school physics, are the smallest components of all matter and are composed of particles called protons, neutrons, and electrons. Atoms of elements can join with atoms of other elements to form molecules.

When an atom is unstable—that is, when its electrons can break off from the nucleus—the electrons give off energy called *radiation*. At the end of the nineteenth century, a physicist named Wilhelm Conrad Roentgen discovered this phenomenon by forcing a flow of electrons through a vacuum tube, which caused a nearby container of a chemical to glow. He called what happened the x-ray because he didn't know what caused it. Several years later, he discovered that the radiation emanating from the vacuum tube could pass through solid objects and leave an impression on a photographic plate. In a flight of fancy, Roentgen placed his wife's hand on a plate and subjected it to the rays—the first x-ray of the human body.

The first medical use of radiation occurred in 1898 when Marie and Pierre Curie discovered an element that gave off radiation naturally. They called it *radium* and saw that it could cause burning. This led to experiments of how radium could be used to affect human cells to treat disease, the first one of which was skin cancer.

In the early 1950s, radioactive cobalt, an artificial isotope (an element that is chemically identical to another element but that differs in atomic weight and electric charge) that can deliver radiation deep into the body without much skin burning, made radiation therapy more practical and effective. In the 1960s, higher-energy machines were developed so that radiation could penetrate even deeper—again with less skin burning.

Types of Radiation

The electromagnetic spectrum is divided into x-rays, ultraviolet rays, and visible light, all of which are forms of energy that consist of particles called *photons*. Different electromagnetic rays have characteristic wavelengths and wave frequencies (the frequency with which waves repeat their patterns). The shorter the waves, the more frequently they repeat and the more energy they have. X-rays have shorter wavelengths and thus higher frequency and more energy than visible light.

Heavy particle radiation uses neutrons or protons, the other two (much heavier) parts of an atom, instead of electrons. It is produced in a device called a *cyclotron*, which creates a much more precise beam than an x-ray.

Neutron beams are characteristically different from x-rays and are sometimes used when a tumor is resistant to X-radiation, such as tumors in the prostate and salivary glands.

Producing and Delivering Radiation

Radiation is produced by a machine called a *linear accelerator*, which is actually a power plant. The machine accelerates electrons, which bounce off a metal target and produce x-rays. The faster the electrons move, the higher the energy of x-rays produced. When the metal target is removed, the x-ray beam is aimed at your tumor.

Dividing a dose of radiation is called *fractionation*. Just as chemotherapy is given in cycles to allow blood cells to repair and replenish themselves, the total dose of radiation is given in parts so that the most possible damage is done to cancer cells while allowing normal cells to recover or be replenished. A full course of radiation treatment is given five days a week and lasts two to eight weeks, for a total of 10 to 40 treatments. During the course of treatment, the radiation is delivered to the same part of the body, but it may be given from different directions in order to minimize skin damage.

Radiation Therapy

There are several ways to use radiation as cancer treatment:

➤ As primary therapy (also called first-line treatment) in some cancers, such as early Hodgkin's disease, some lung cancers, and head and neck cancer
➤ Used alone as a cure or combined with surgery and/or chemotherapy
➤ As palliation—that is, to relieve symptoms rather than cure the disease

Low-energy x-rays, such as dental and chest x-rays, pass harmlessly through your body and are used for diagnosis. *High-energy x-rays* are capable of penetrating the body and are used for radiation therapy. Because they damage all of the cells they contact, radiation therapy does carry side effects; although only tumor cells are the "real" targets of the radiation, tissue immediately adjacent to the tumor also is irradiated.

High-energy radiation interacts with cell molecules and damages vital structures such as DNA or cellular enzymes. Some tumor cells are killed outright, and some are so damaged that they cannot reproduce and therefore will also die eventually. Cells are most vulnerable when they are actively dividing, so, as with most chemotherapeutic drugs, radiation therapy is most effective on dividing cells. This is why radiation therapy is given in fractions over a period of time—as is chemotherapy. In addition, as the tumor shrinks, each of the cells receives more oxygen, which makes them even more vulnerable to the effects of radiation. The less oxygen a cell contains, the more radiation it takes to kill it.

External Radiation

There are two general ways to deliver radiation: externally and internally. When the source of radiation comes from outside your body—that is, from a linear accelerator or other device—it is called *external beam irradiation*. There are two major types of external beam radiation. *Orthovoltage* radiation does not penetrate deeply and is used to treat surface tumors such as skin cancer. *Megavoltage* (also called high-energy) radiation is used to treat most other cancers because it is strong enough to penetrate deep tumors. It is often directed at the tumor from more than one location.

The radiation does its job on the tumor and then passes out of your body. In order to provide maximum tumor penetration and to minimize irradiation of healthy tissue, the beam of radiation is placed very precisely by means of diagnostic scans and computers. The radiation oncologist will use marking pens so the technician will know exactly where to focus the beam, and this is why you are cautioned not to move during the treatment. To help you stay still, they will cushion your body and support it with plaster or foam devices.

Intraoperative radiation therapy (IORT) is given during surgery. An external beam radiation machine with a special adapter is brought into the operating room, and a large dose of radiation is delivered to the tumor. This creates a significantly decreased risk of damaging healthy tissue. IORT also can be used as prophylaxis at the tumor site after a tumor has been removed in order to destroy cells that may have been released into the bloodstream as a result of the surgery.

Stereotactic radiation therapy, now used almost exclusively for brain cancer, targets a tumor from a number of different directions so that beams of radiation converge. This technique, which is controlled by computer, ensures that a sufficient total amount of radiation is delivered to the tumor, but the amount of exposure to surrounding tissues is minimized. CT scans and MRI imaging map the precise location of the tumor, and the patient's head is held absolutely still by means of a clamping device. It is sometimes possible to avoid brain surgery with stereotactic radiation.

Internal Radiation

When the source of radiation comes from inside your body, it is called *brachytherapy*—and yes, you are radioactive for a period of time. Brachytherapy involves placing a source of radiation enclosed in a container, such as a needle or tube, close to the tumor. The source is called a *radioisotope*. The element iridium is usually the source, but it might also be cesium, iodine, phosphorus, or gold. The placement is done by a computer and the radioisotope is removed immediately after the treatment, which usually lasts only about 10 minutes. Radioisotopes also can be injected into the bloodstream, where they head directly for the tumor. The dose is fractionated. Methods of brachytherapy delivery include the following:

➤ *Interstitial radiation* therapy means that the radiation implant, filled with radioactive seeds, is placed directly into the tumor and surrounding tissue. The implants remain in place for three to five days, during which time the radioisotope decays, giving off less and less radiation. Depending on the type of implant, it is either removed or left in place permanently.

➤ *Intercavitary* therapy is placement of a hollow container inside a body cavity like the uterus or vagina. The radioactive source is *afterloaded* (inserted into the container after the container is inserted into the body) and left in place for two to three days. Then the entire container is removed.

➤ *Intraluminal* radiation therapy delivers radiation to the opening (lumen) of hollow organs (such as the esophagus), and the container is placed near the tumor. The radioactive source is then afterloaded.

➤ *High-dose rate remote afterloading* is similar to other types of brachytherapy except that the radiation source is not loaded manually. Instead, a machine delivers it through a specially designed conduit, and because of the unusually high dose, it is left in place for hours instead of days. This procedure is done on an outpatient rather than inpatient basis.

Total Radiation

Total body irradiation (TBI) is just what it sounds like: irradiation of the entire body to destroy distant metastases that are not detectable on various scans. It is used most commonly in preparation for bone marrow transplantation (see Chapter 5) instead of, or in addition to, high-dose chemotherapy. A variation of TBI is *total lymphoid irradiation*, in which only lymph nodes are irradiated and the rest of the body is shielded. TBI is done once or twice a day for several days prior to the transplant.

Pros and Cons of Radiation Therapy

As with all types of cancer treatment, radiation therapy has advantages and disadvantages. Because it has no effect on distant metastases, it is most effective when used on a tumor in situ—that is, one that has not advanced or metastasized. It can kill tumors without disfiguring the patient (as in head and neck cancer) and without significant damage to healthy adjacent tissue. Because different types of tumors vary widely in terms of *radiosensitivity*, radiation therapy is not effective for all cancers.

Treatment is given by a *radiation oncologist*, who is a medical subspecialist, and when you are referred to this physician, he or she will probably take a detailed history and review your treatment to date. Much of the success of radiation therapy results from the skill of the radiation oncologist and radiation technicians, and because radiation oncology combines medicine and technology, it is a rapidly changing field. In addition, even though much of the procedure has become standardized, you still ought to check out the credentials and experience of the people who will be prescribing and administering your radiation therapy.

Preparation for Radiation Therapy

Preparation for radiotherapy involves determining the precise area of your body (the treatment field) that will be irradiated and the position you will have to assume during the treatment. This is called *simulation* and takes two or three hours. The radiation oncologist will determine which of several irradiation techniques will be used, the dose of the radiation therapy, and the fractionation. After the precise positioning has been determined, your skin will be marked with ink and the radiation site will be recorded with x-rays. Or you might be tattooed—not with a snarling dragon or the name of your honey inside a heart, but with a tiny black dot that has the advantage of permanence. You can think of it as a souvenir of successful treatment.

A medical or *radiation physicist* helps plan the treatment and is responsible for the equipment. Upon receiving instructions from the radiation oncologist, a *dosimetrist* calculates the amount of radiation you will receive and how long each treatment will last. A *technologist* positions you and actually operates the equipment, and you may also be seen by a *radiation nurse*.

If this seems like a lot of people involved in your treatment, it is—but you should see the crowd in the operating room! Seriously though, radiation therapy is a highly precise and highly technical form of cancer treatment, and each health professional's skill is different from each other's. Together they form a smooth team—with you, of course, as the star player.

Side Effects of Radiation Therapy

Although radiation therapy is generally safe and effective, as with any other medical treatment, there are a number of side effects, almost all of which are temporary but may take a while to heal. Also, the nature of the side effects depends on the part of the body irradiated, and their severity is a function of the dose of radiation. For those side effects that are similar to chemotherapy, refer to Chapter 7 for ways to cope with and minimize them.

➤ *Fatigue.* As with chemotherapy, fatigue is the most common side effect. The larger the area being irradiated, the more likely it is that fatigue will occur. It begins early and increases throughout the course of treatment, peaking during the third to fifth weeks. Although no one knows why fatigue so often accompanies radiation therapy, some of the probable causes include: depletion of energy as a result of the healing process; buildup of toxic waste as cells are killed; increased metabolism; and the effort required to make daily trips to the hospital.

➤ *Anorexia.* Many people suffer from anorexia, a loss of appetite, because cell changes may affect the way hunger signals are sent to the brain or because there are changes in the sense of taste. Also, the stress of being sick and the fatigue and tedium of having to go to the hospital every day can take away one's appetite very quickly.

➤ *Skin reactions.* Dermatitis is common because the beam of radiation passes through the skin on its way to the tumor. If you've ever had a sunburn, you'll know what radiation dermatitis looks and feels like. Your skin may feel dry, itchy, flaky, and flushed, or it may darken. Don't be surprised if the skin opposite the site of the treated area also develops a reaction. This is called *exit dermatitis* and is a result of the

radiation leaving your body. If possible, the radiation oncologist will try to minimize dermatitis by approaching the
tumor from more than one direction, and there are a
number of things you can do for yourself: avoid exposure to
the sun (put at least SPF 15 sun block on *every time* you go
outdoors—not just in summer—and wear a hat with a wide
brim if it's sunny); don't use skin products that contain
alcohol (some colognes and aftershave lotion) because they
are very drying; wear soft fabrics that won't irritate skin;
don't swim in chlorinated pools or soak in a hot tub; take a
warm or cool bath or shower instead of a hot one; use a
moisturizing lotion that contains aloe vera, which is very
soothing, or sprinkle cornstarch on skin folds. If the dermatitis is very severe, your physician will prescribe a med-
icated ointment.

➤ *Local reactions.* These are very common. For example, mouth
soreness and/or extreme dryness of the mouth and lips often
accompany radiation of the head and neck. Nausea is an
infrequent complication of radiation therapy and usually
occurs only when the stomach and brain are irradiated. Why
the brain? Because that's where the vomiting center is
located, and it is easily stimulated by radiation.

➤ *Diarrhea.* This often accompanies abdominal radiation
because the cells of the intestine divide rapidly and are thus
highly vulnerable to radiation. They also react to radiation
by producing more water and mucous, which you experience
as desperate trips to the bathroom.

➤ *Hair loss.* You may lose some hair a few weeks after radiation
therapy. The reasons for hair loss are the same as with
chemotherapy, but the pattern of loss is different. Your entire
crop of body hair won't fall out, but you will have bald
patches wherever the radiation enters and exits your body.
These may be permanent or temporary.

➤ *Inflammation of the bladder.* If you have radiation treatment
for bladder cancer, cancer of the reproductive organs or
prostate, or anywhere in the pelvis, you may get *cystitis*
(inflammation of the bladder). Symptoms include feeling that
your bladder is full when it isn't, the urge to urinate frequently, and burning and/or bleeding on urination. This is a

temporary condition, but while you have symptoms, you should increase fluid intake so your urine is not so concentrated. You also may get a prescription for Pyridium, which is a bladder anesthetic.

➤ *Bowel obstructions.* A very small number of people (about 2 percent) who receive pelvic or abdominal irradiation get a bowel obstruction, which can occur months or even years after treatment. The major symptoms are pain and nausea with retching, and it requires emergency surgery.

➤ *Coughing/shortness of breath.* Breast irradiation sometimes causes chronic coughing or shortness of breath because lungs may be damaged. Depending on the angle of the beam and the location of the tumor, a portion of a lung may have been exposed to radiation.

In addition to these temporary effects, there are two major long-term effects of radiation therapy. Treatment to the pelvic area may result in decreased fertility and possibly sterility (the permanent inability to reproduce). Women may stop menstruating and have trouble becoming pregnant, and men may suffer from decreased sperm production and motility—and thus diminished ability to impregnate. Some men also will become impotent. *Women receiving radiation should be very careful not to become pregnant before and during the course of the treatment because serious fetal damage can occur.* Since the radiation doesn't linger, they may begin trying to conceive soon after the treatments have ended, but they should first speak with their doctor.

A phenomenon that carries irony to its outer limits is that sometimes radiation therapy causes cancer. Since low doses of radiation have been known to increase the risk of cancer in some people, it is reasonable to assume that therapeutic doses, which are much higher, make the risk that much worse. Still, even though risk exists, it is very low and is not a logical reason to refuse radiation therapy as a treatment for an existing cancer. To put it another way, not treating an existing cancer with radiation (if that is the most effective therapy) creates a far greater risk than the possibility of a second cancer a decade or so later.

The most common radiation-induced cancer is leukemia, which occurs 5 to 10 years after treatment. Thyroid and breast cancers and sarcomas can appear 15 years after treatment. In addition, the younger people are when they are irradiated (and the greater the body surface exposed), the higher the risk of a second, radiation-induced, cancer.

Surgery

A majority of cancer patients have surgery at one time or another during the course of diagnosis and treatment. It usually takes the form of a biopsy or an operation to remove the tumor.

Surgery alone as a cure for cancer is effective only when a solid tumor is small and completely localized. The object is to remove the entire tumor and a small amount of healthy tissue surrounding it (called the *margin*).

When there is either evidence or a strong likelihood of metastasis, surgery is used to remove as much of the tumor as possible, and then treatment is continued with adjuvant chemotherapy or radiation. Pretreatment with chemotherapy or radiation also can be used prior to surgery to shrink the tumor and make it easier to see and remove.

The problem with using surgery alone is that it is never possible to say with absolute certainty that a sufficient number of cancer cells have not broken off from the tumor and slid into the bloodstream to establish metastases. In many types of cancer—such as colorectal, lung, malignant melanoma, brain tumors, and the like—adjuvant chemotherapy is used routinely following surgery.

Other reasons to operate on cancer patients include: removal of metastases; palliation of symptoms such as intestinal or other block-ages; relief of intractable pain by severing nerves; implantation of radioactive elements; restoration of body parts previously disfigured by surgery (for example, breast reconstruction); and implantation of intravenous ports for long-term administration of chemotherapy.

A Short History

Surgery to treat cancer has a long and checkered history. Records from ancient Egypt as early as 1600 B.C.E. tell of tumors being removed—without benefit of anesthesia, of course, and without ben-efit of much knowledge about the nature of cancer. Some patients actually survived, though, and lived for a while.

In the early nineteenth century, surgical treatment of cancer began in earnest when Ephraim McDowell, a Kentucky physician, removed an ovarian tumor that weighed more than 20 pounds. The operation was surprisingly successful because the woman lived through it—again, without benefit of anesthesia. She didn't die until 30 years later.

Battlefield surgery, mostly amputations, has been practiced for centuries. In the beginning, surgeons were barbers (hence the traditional red and white barber pole which represented the flow of blood from the barbers' sideline practice). These barbers were noted more for the speed of their operations than for the finesse of their surgical skill. Speed was crucial (it is still an important factor) because there was no anesthesia and no antibiotics.

However, when Florence Nightingale, a British nurse, went to the Crimea in the 1850s to care for soldiers wounded in the Crimean War, she insisted on cleanliness (frequent handwashing, cleaning of instruments, and the like) and adequate nutrition. As a result, there were far fewer wound infections than had been common up until then. Unfortunately, her principles of hygiene did not cross the Atlantic Ocean to be put into practice in hospital tents during the American Civil War, and more soldiers from both sides died of infection than from gunshot wounds.

After 1846, when Morton first used general anesthesia to remove a cancerous tumor of the mouth, surgery began to be thought of as a practical option for treating cancer. Then, in the late nineteenth century, when the principles of antisepsis came into somewhat common use, surgery turned into an even more viable option because patients were less likely to die of massive infection—after surviving the operation itself. Joseph Lister had convinced surgeons to wash their hands as well as their instruments before operating, and surgical instruments that helped stem blood loss came into common use. In addition, discovery of the microscope made cancer surgery a viable treatment option.

At the end of the nineteenth century, William Halsted, known as the father of American surgery, after studying in Germany and Austria, brought advanced surgical techniques to the United States, and he taught the importance of careful laboratory investigation before operating. At the same time in Germany, Rudolf Virchow discovered the cellular basis of tissue growth and repair—and as a result, the nature of wound healing. He and his colleagues on both sides of the Atlantic were responsible for the modern study of pathology, and the gradual fading in medical circles of belief in evil or noxious humors as the cause of disease.

At the time that Halsted was operating and teaching in New York City, cancer patients always waited until their tumors were large and far advanced before submitting to the surgeon's scalpel. And who could blame them? Surgery was still a pretty primitive endeavor, and the mortality rate was high. Halsted, however, advocated radical surgery as soon as the tumor was discovered, and his most lasting contribution (many women refer to it as an infamous contribution) to the art of surgery was the Halsted procedure to cure breast cancer in which the entire breast, as well as adjacent lymph nodes and the surrounding muscle tissue, were removed. It was a terribly disfiguring operation—but it cured many cases of breast cancer.

Surgery today is highly sophisticated, and a modern operating room has some of the aura of a spaceship. Scalpels and sutures are still used, but they are no longer a surgeon's only instrument; he or she uses lasers to "cut" into organs, stapling devices to close wounds, minuscule cameras to peer into closed spaces, and a wide variety of invasive and noninvasive monitoring devices to measure all body functions during and after the procedure.

In addition, there have been major improvements in postoperative care, including infection prevention, pain control, replacement of lost fluids and nutrients, and a deeper understanding of how surgery affects all body systems.

Type and Extent of Surgery

The type of surgery, the body part on which it takes place, and the extent of tissue removed (*resected*) all play a role in how you will react to and recover from the operation. There are a number of types of surgery that cancer patients undergo:

> *Preventive surgery* to remove precancerous lesions such as polyps is very common. It is called *prophylactic*, is usually done under local anesthesia, and is considered a minor operation (although an old medical adage says that "minor" is what the surgeon does and "major" is what the patient experiences).

Other examples of prophylactic surgery include removal of all or part of the colon because of ulcerative colitis, and mastectomy for women at very high risk of breast cancer, a procedure that is highly controversial.

➤ *Biopsy* is performed for diagnosis and staging (see Chapter 1). Sometimes surgery is the only way to visualize the extent of the tumor and, to some extent, to determine the amount of metastasis. Staging surgery is done either by *laparotomy* (opening the abdomen) or *laparoscopy* (inserting a laparascope, a long, thin scoping device, with fiberoptic bundle attached) to view abdominal contents through a very small incision.

➤ *Second-look surgery*, also called *retreatment* staging, allows the surgeon to see how successful treatment has been, and to examine the organs and tissues in and around the primary site.

➤ *Treatment surgery* involves resecting (removing) diseased tissue as well as normal-appearing tissue that surrounds it: the margin, as in "margin of safety." As a rule, nearby lymph nodes are examined for metastasis and removed if they are found to be malignant or simply if they are too close to the tumor site. In order to prevent disfigurement, surgeons try to remove as little tissue as is safely possible, and then use adjuvant radiotherapy or chemotherapy to kill distant metastases and/or cancer cells that escaped during the operation.

➤ *Cytoreductive surgery* may take place if a tumor is so large and the cancer so far advanced that it cannot be cured. With cytoreductive surgery, a surgeon removes as much of the tumor as possible without causing a permanent loss of organ function. Cytoreductive surgery is followed by radiation and/or chemotherapy. It is almost never curative and is done only if there's a reasonable chance that the tumor can be successfully treated by other means.

Surgery may take place to remove a secondary tumor that is not responding to chemotherapy after the primary tumor has been completely removed.

➤ *Emergency surgery* may be necessary if the tumor has caused internal or external hemorrhage, intestinal or respiratory obstruction, or other threats that must be corrected immediately.

➤ *Palliative surgery* is done to relieve symptoms (such as reducing a lung cancer that has grown so large it interferes with breathing); improve quality of life (such as *debulking* a tumor so that it does not impinge on sensory nerves); or implant various devices that aid in assisting life (such as inserting a gastric feeding tube). It is not intended to be curative.

➤ *Reconstructive surgery* (also called *rehabilitative* surgery) is designed to reconstruct tissues after major disfiguring surgery, such as breast reconstruction following mastectomy.

Surgery to implant pumps, catheters, and other devices to administer drugs and radioisotopes may be done to support chemotherapy and radiation. (See Chapter 2 for a discussion of these devices.)

The Surgical Experience

Many people, by the time they reach adulthood, have had surgery (perhaps a tonsillectomy or appendectomy in their youth) and are somewhat familiar with the procedure. But not everyone has, and because the technology and procedures change so fast, what follows will be a brief description of an abdominal operation. This may not be exactly what you will experience, but it is representative of surgery in general. Also, you might want to do some reading or other research before your operation.

Preparation for Abdominal Surgery

Since your insurance company won't allow you to be admitted to the hospital the night before your operation (unless you are already there receiving other treatment), you'll have to spend a few hours there the week before to have your preoperative tests: blood work, urinalysis, electrocardiogram, and chest x-ray. If you want to bank a few units of blood for yourself, or ask a friend with the same blood type to donate for you, call the hospital blood bank about six weeks before your scheduled operation and inquire about the procedure. If you bank two units, for example, you usually have to begin about a month before the procedure.

If you smoke, you will be told to stop about a month before surgery (and if you can last that long without a cigarette, you can and should quit altogether). Respiratory problems are the most common and serious postoperative complication, and their incidence and severity are greatly increased if you smoke.

In cancer surgery, although you don't have a great deal of lead time, as soon as you find out you'll need an operation, you should begin eating as well as possible and pay particular attention to increasing your protein intake (proteins are one of the major factors in tissue repair). Get some exercise before you go into the hospital. This does not mean becoming an overnight jock, but there's no reason why you can't go for a long, brisk walk every day before surgery to increase your stamina.

Some time before, or perhaps on the day of surgery, you will be required to sign a consent form. Read it carefully and make certain you know exactly what you're giving permission for. You should have discussed all the ramifications of the operation before you get down to the final consent, but there still may be questions in your mind. If so, don't be shy about asking. This is *your* body.

On the day of the operation, you'll be told to check into the hospital a few hours before your operation is scheduled. (Surgeons are morning people, so you'll probably have to show up by 5:00 or 6:00 A.M.) You'll change into a gown, and either your clothes will be put into a bag and sent to your room, or whoever comes to the hospital with you can take them home. By the way, leave *all* your jewelry and valuables at home. A visitor can bring your watch, eyeglasses, and a few dollars for the newspaper or candy the next day. You won't need any of that stuff while you're on the operating table.

When you have donned that darling little hospital gown, you'll be weighed. (It's for the anesthesia, but you don't have to look at the scale!) Then you'll lie on a stretcher, and a nurse will start an intravenous infusion (or this might not be done until you are actually on the operating table). The nurse will also take your blood pressure, and probably ask many of the same questions you've answered a dozen times already. Shortly, you'll be taken to the operating suite. Before you're actually taken into the room where the deed will be done, your surgeon will stop by to say hello. This is the time to speak up if you have last-minute questions, or if you have changed your mind about the surgery.

This is also the time when your anesthesiologist will speak with you if you haven't already met him or her. The anesthesiologist will ask about your past experiences with anesthesia and about your drug allergies. *Always* insist on a board-certified anesthesiologist (a physician). Do this two or three days prior to the operation. Do not allow a nurse anesthetist (who is not a physician) to give you anesthesia unless that person is attended by an anesthesiologist in the operating room *the entire time* you are under anesthesia.

Not long after your surgeon has said good-bye and gone off to scrub, you'll be wheeled into the actual operating room (O.R.) and be told to scoot over from the stretcher to the operating table (which will look impossibly narrow and you'll be certain that you can't fit—but you can). If you have never been in an O.R. before, take some time to look around and ask questions if you want. In the first place, it's very interesting (although not as dramatic as it appears on television), and second, looking at the instruments and machines will take your mind off your nervousness. And you *will* be nervous. It doesn't matter how blasé you are or how many times you have had surgery, being cut open and having someone poke around among your innards is a nerve-wracking experience. If you don't feel like looking around or talking with the nurses, try lying quietly and breathing deeply to relax.

You won't have much time to worry or chat, because very soon after you are strapped to the operating table (for your safety, just like car seat belts), you will receive a dose of a very fast-acting analgesic. (This is not the general anesthesia; that's given to you after you're asleep.) Alternately, you may be asked to sit on the edge of the table while the anesthesiologist inserts the needle for spinal anesthesia. The needle for the analgesic is pushed into your IV tube rather than into your skin, so you may not know it's going to happen. That's the last you will be aware of until you wake up in the recovery room, so if you don't want to be caught unawares—or if you want to say a little prayer, perhaps—ask the anesthesiologist to let you know before you get the jolt of analgesia. Otherwise, once it's in your bloodstream, you won't know what hit you.

Regarding anesthesia, there are three major types:

➤ *Local anesthesia* is given by needle and temporarily deadens a small area of tissue. You remain awake. This is the type dentists use when you get a shot of novocaine before a filling or root canal. *Topical anesthesia* is a type of local, but it is sprayed or painted onto the surface of the skin or mucous membrane.

➤ *Regional anesthesia*, also called *nerve block*, blocks sensation to a larger area of the body. It is injected into the spinal fluid in the lower back and numbs you from the pelvic region down to the bottom of your feet. Depending on how long the operation is to last, it can be given in a single injection or as a continuous infusion. Also, depending on the nature of the surgery and its length, you may have only regional anesthesia, in which case you remain awake but heavily sedated, or regional anesthesia combined with a general, in which case you are asleep.

➤ *General anesthesia* means that you are not only asleep but in a kind of suspended animation. The anesthesia is administered as a gas through a face mask after you have been given the fast-acting analgesia, and it renders you incapable of any sensation at all.

After an Abdominal Operation

When you wake up from the anesthesia, you will be in pain. After all, you've just been subjected to a big knife wound. The good news is that it doesn't last long (by the end of the second or third day, you probably won't need narcotics), and the pain medication you will receive really works.

There's a wonderful new tool in the postoperative pain medication armamentarium: *patient-controlled analgesia* (PCA). The surgeon hooks this up to your IV right in the O.R., and it consists of premeasured doses of morphine, Demerol, or another drug. You give yourself a dose of analgesia by pushing a little button on a small computer, also attached to the IV tubing. This lets you medicate yourself when you need it (push the button before the pain reaches white-hot intensity so the morphine takes less time to act on the pain and is more effective); you don't have to ask the nurses, who may forget about you because they're so busy; and you usually end up needing smaller doses less frequently because you're getting the morphine intravenously rather than intramuscularly (a shot in the butt). And don't worry: you can't overdose. The system is automatically programmed to shut itself off when the preset dose has gone into your vein.

PCA can also be given *intrathecally*—into your spinal canal via a very small plastic catheter. It works the same way: you push a button and a dose of fentanyl, morphine, or other drug flows into the cerebrospinal fluid. Sometimes a local anesthetic such as lidocaine or a similar drug is mixed in with the fentanyl and may cause numbness in one of your legs so that you'll have difficulty standing and walking. This will disappear when the intrathecal catheter is removed, but if it makes you nervous, ask to have it taken out and to receive PCA through the IV in your arm.

There's no doubt that you'll feel fairly rotten for the rest of the day of abdominal surgery. You'll be allowed to drink sips of clear fluids, and the nurses will make you get up to go to the bathroom (unless you have an indwelling urinary catheter, which will remain in place for a day or two). Getting up may hurt like blazes, but do it anyway because the sooner you're on your feet and shuffling around, the faster you will heal and the better you will feel. And it's about a thousand times better than using a bedpan.

The next morning you'll be hungry, since you haven't eaten since the night before the operation. Your IV may be disconnected that day or the day after (although the needle with a little plastic stopper attached will remain in your arm until you go home). You'll probably want to comb your hair, shave, or put on a dab of lipstick. By the following day, you'll be walking in the hospital corridors. (If it hurts, stand up as straight as you can and force yourself to do it even if the nurses don't make you.) You'll also be eating real food, reading your novel, and nagging your surgeon about taking a shower and going home. But stay in the hospital as long as your insurance company will let you, because when you get home, you won't have the advantages of a hospital bed with its side rails to help you get in and out, and you probably won't have people to wait on you.

You may have some complications, either immediately after the abdominal surgery, a day or so later, or when you get home. The most common is a wound infection, which is serious but treatable with IV antibiotics. Rarely, you could have bleeding from the incision or internal bleeding, which also is serious and might necessitate another trip to the O.R. Postoperative pneumonia or a blood clot in a vein are hardly ever seen anymore because patients get out of bed and move around very soon after surgery. But they do occur once in a while, and both need to be treated in the hospital.

An incisional infection has to be opened and drained. This is not as uncommon as hospitals would like it to be (it is *always* a hospital-contracted infection and even has its own medical term: *nosocomial infection*), but it always resolves itself with antibiotics and time. However, if the wound has to be opened (the stitches or staples removed), it is not surgically closed again. Rather, it is allowed to heal by itself from the inside out. This is called healing by *granulation*. The procedure looks unappealing (because the wound is raw and red and open and you can see into it), but it doesn't hurt because the skin and muscle nerves were severed during surgery and take several months to regenerate—long after the incision has healed.

Once you're up and about, your bowel function will return to normal, but the first bowel movement can be pretty uncomfortable because your abdominal muscles may not be up to the task. Ask your doctor to prescribe a stool softener (like Colace), or bring your own to the hospital and take one a day beginning the day of surgery.

There are a few other complications you need to be aware of, some more common than others and some more serious than others: kidney or bladder infection; hemorrhage, sometimes requiring transfusion; blood clots; and death, brain damage, or paralysis from anesthesia.

Surgery Without Sharp Instruments

Not all operations involve cutting into the body with a scalpel. Sometimes, with all the high-tech equipment, an operating room looks more like the control room of a spaceship than a place where medical procedures are going on.

Laser Treatment

Practically everyone knows someone who has had laser therapy—for cataracts or to have a growth on the skin removed. And there's almost no one in the United States who hasn't seen the laser duel between Darth Vader and Luke Skywalker in *Star Wars*. So the word *laser* is part of everyone's vocabulary, but few people really know what it means—and how it can be used to treat cancer.

LASER is an acronym for *light amplification by stimulated emission of radiation*. It was first patented in 1957 by Gordon Gould, and the first working model was built around 1960. Essentially a laser is a beam of light highly concentrated in an enclosed space. As the light is produced, it is further amplified by substances contained in the laser tube. These substances include gases such as carbon dioxide, argon, and neodymium:yttrium-aluminum-garnet (NdYAG).

In surgery, the laser beam is used to cut and vaporize tissue, and it is often superior to a scalpel because there is minimal bleeding. Because the beam can be focused with great precision, it is often used for *microsurgery*—that is, surgery that takes place in very small places, like the eye. Two of the most common types of laser surgery include:

➤ *Endoscopic*, in which a laser beam is sent through a flexible tube called an *endoscope*. An endoscope can be passed through any opening in the body: anus, mouth, vagina, or nose. The person doing the procedure can look through the scope and aim the laser beam at whatever needs to be removed, usually a polyp or other small growth. It is technically possible to remove tumors this way, but it is not usually done (unless the tumor is very small and very well defined) because the laser can't penetrate below the visible surface of the tumor, where more cancer cells are probably lurking. The exception is tumors of the trachea, which can't be successfully treated with regular surgery. Even so, several laser treatments are required because the tumor will most likely grow back.
➤ *Photodynamic laser therapy* involves injecting a chemical called hematoporphyrin prior to the laser procedure. Hematoporphyrin makes certain tissue, such as some types of malignancies, in the mouth, for example, more sensitive to light.

Hyperthermia

Hyperthermia means elevated temperature, and in cancer treatment, it refers to the use of heat to kill cancer cells. The treatment is still investigational, and the theory is that cancer cells do not tolerate heat as well as normal cells. It is not used by itself but rather as an adjuvant treatment with chemotherapy or radiotherapy because heat may make cancer cells more sensitive to these two treatment modalities. Hyperthermia is especially effective when used with radiotherapy because two types of cells are resistant to radiotherapy: those manufacturing DNA as they prepare for cell division, and those that are poorly oxygenated.

Hyperthermia has been used to beneficial effect in chest wall recurrences of breast cancer, metastatic melanoma in the skin and nearby lymph nodes, cervical cancer, bladder cancer, and cancers of the lip and mouth.

When tissue is heated above 106° F, cells begin to die, which is why it is so dangerous not to bring down a high fever. The degree of damage depends on the amount of heat and the length of time it is applied. Temperatures used in treating cancer with hyperthermia range from 106° to 133°F.

Hyperthermia sounds a little scary—as if you were going to be cooked like a lobster. It's not bad at all, although sometimes it hurts. Heating localized tumors on or near the surface of the body is done by an external applicator that has a connected heat source (such as a microwave, radio frequency, or ultrasound). Localized tumors also can be heated from within (called *interstitial hyperthermia*) by inserting a plastic tube with a needle while you are under local anesthesia. The heat source is then inserted directly into the tube through the needle. The advantage of interstitial hyperthermia is that temperatures can be raised much higher than by going through the skin, and there is much less damage to surrounding tissues.

Regional hyperthermia uses microwave or radio frequency applicators to heat large amounts of tissue deep inside the body, and *external whole-body hyperthermia* is done by means of hot water blankets or devices that look like ovens. *Internal whole-body hyperthermia* means that the patient's blood is removed, heated, and then returned to the body—not all at once, of course. Since temperatures cannot be elevated to more than 108°F, whole-body may not be particularly effective. This technique is still highly investigational and is used only for deep tumors or liquid tumors.

Hyperthermia does not potentiate any of the side effects of chemotherapy or radiation therapy, but superficial treatment can cause discomfort, pain, blisters (which heal quickly), and possibly burns (which do not heal quickly and may require plastic surgery to repair).

Cryosurgery

Cryosurgery is the opposite of hyperthermia. Here you're sent to the freezer instead of the microwave oven! Seriously—cryosurgery (also called *cryotherapy*) means applying extreme cold to freeze tissue.

It is essentially frostbite—which is commonly known to damage tissue if serious enough—that is carried to an extreme, and done under medically controlled conditions.

Cryosurgery as a treatment for cancer consists of placing refrigeration agents (liquid nitrogen or argon gas) contained in a hollow vacuum-insulated tube or probe inside or next to tumors to destroy them. The tissue is frozen to -320°F. It then thaws and is left inside the body to form scar tissue. Surface tumors are left to form a scab, which eventually falls off and may leave a scar depending on the depth and size of the tumor.

Major advantages of cryosurgery are that it minimizes damage to surrounding tissue, and there is less bleeding. Even if large blood vessels are frozen, they are not harmed because the flow of warm blood protects them. The disadvantages are that an open surgical procedure is required to reach deep tumors, and there are some rare side effects: increase in white blood cell count and temperature elevation that usually resolve quickly; hemorrhage after liver cryosurgery; infection; temporary urinary incontinence after cryosurgery on the prostate; and fluid retention in the lungs. One not-so-minor side effect is the strong likelihood of impotence after prostate freezing because the frozen area extends beyond the prostate itself to tissues that contain nerves that control erection. The impotence may or may not be permanent, so it is something to think about before agreeing to the procedure.

Cryosurgery is currently used for primary and metastatic tumors of the liver and prostate, as well as some bone cancers and gynecologic cancers. Not all cancer patients are good candidates for cryosurgery. A CT scan or an MRI is used to assess the size and location of the tumor, and then the following criteria are applied:

> The patient should be in relatively good general health with intact liver function (if liver cancer is the issue).
> The tumor must be such that conventional surgery is not appropriate.
> If the patient has been treated with surgery and/or chemotherapy, and the tumor has shrunk but the disease itself has not been cured, cryosurgery may be a good next choice.

> Liver cryosurgery is used when the original tumor was successfully removed but there is concern that some tumor cells remain in the margin. A flat probe is then used to freeze the cut edge of the liver.
> Someone with multiple tumors can benefit from having the largest removed surgically and the others frozen.

Surgery for Specific Cancers

As you read about the following types of operations for various cancers, keep one thing in mind: the amount and kind of surgery that might cure the disease or put it into long-term remission depends entirely on the stage. It also depends on other factors such as your general health at the time of diagnosis, other accompanying illnesses, the degree and location of metastasis, and other cancer treatments you have had prior to surgery.

Moreover, these descriptions are only a general guide to the operations most usually done. Your surgeon will describe to you the specifics of your surgery. Remember that you can ask for as much or as little detail as you feel comfortable knowing.

Adrenal Glands

The adrenal glands are small organs sitting atop the kidneys that secrete various hormones. There are two types of adrenal malignancy, both very rare: adrenocortical cancer and pheochromocytoma.

> The adrenal gland is removed, along with malignant tissue that surrounds it in the kidney and liver. Surgery is followed by adjuvant chemotherapy.

Anus

The anus is the outlet of the bowel and lies at the lower end of the rectum. Anal cancer, which is rare and very curable, is almost always squamous cell carcinoma. A combination of radiation and chemotherapy may be curative, which is the goal to preserve function of the sphincter, the circular muscle that allows you to control your bowels.

➤ *Abdominoperineal resection* is removal of the rectum and anus for advanced disease and results in a temporary or permanent *colostomy* (an opening in the abdominal wall through which feces pass into an attached plastic bag).

➤ If the cancer is not advanced, only the tumor and a margin is removed, and every effort is made to preserve sphincter function.

Bile Duct

The bile duct is a tube that drains bile from the liver to the small intestine. Cancer of the bile duct is not common, and it is usually not diagnosed until is fairly difficult to cure by surgery alone. Surgery is followed by adjuvant radiotherapy.

➤ If the tumor has not spread to the lymph nodes and is confined to either the left or right duct, it and the accompanying lobe of the liver are removed.

➤ If the tumor is at the junction of the left and right ducts, it is removed, and the bile ducts are rebuilt using a loop of the small intestine.

➤ If the tumor is at the far end of the duct where it empties into the small intestine, radical surgery is necessary. This involves removing part of the intestine and the pancreas. This is extremely complicated surgery and is done only in extreme cases.

Bladder

Bladder cancer is the most frequent cancer of the urinary tract. It rarely develops until middle age and is much more common in men than women. The vast majority of bladder cancer (90 percent) is transitional cell carcinoma, which arises from certain epithelial cells that line the bladder. Other types of the disease include papillary, squamous cell carcinoma, and adenocarcinoma.

➤ *Partial cystectomy*, indicated for a single primary tumor in a patient with no prior history of bladder cancer, involves removing only the cancerous portion of the bladder—with a 2-cm (about ¾-inch) margin of healthy tissue. It is accompanied by adjuvant chemotherapy.

> *Radical cystectomy* for invasive bladder cancer includes removing the entire bladder, surrounding tissue and fat, as well as pelvic lymph nodes. In women, all reproductive organs, as well as the anterior portion of the vagina, also are removed. Men lose their prostate gland and seminal vesicles (structures that store one component of semen).

> *Transurethral resection* (TUR) is a procedure in which a scope is inserted into the bladder and the tumors are burned (*fulgurated*) off. This procedure is used only when the tumor(s) is small, usually less than 2 cm, and easily accessible to the scope. It is accompanied by adjuvant chemotherapy.

Blood Vessels

Kaposi's sarcoma (KS) used to be a very rare cancer of the blood vessels, which occurred almost exclusively in men of Mediterranean descent and people who were immunocompromised. It is now extremely common in people with AIDS, who have a more virulent and aggressive form of the disease. Lesions are both external, which appear as dark red or purple sores, and internal.

> External lesions can be removed surgically, but this is always accompanied, preceded, or followed by adjuvant chemotherapy and/or radiation.

Bone and Soft Tissue

Primary bone cancer is relatively rare and is seen most often in children and adolescents. However, metastasis to the bone from other primary sites (most commonly the breast, lung, and prostate) is very common.

> Radical surgery consists of amputation or excision of the tumor with wide margins. If a muscle is involved, the entire muscle group is excised. If a major blood vessel is involved, then the entire vessel is stripped and replaced with an artificial graft. Even with this much surgery, local recurrence is common; therefore, it is always followed by adjuvant chemotherapy.

> Conservative surgery attempts to spare the limb, and to leave a narrower margin of normal tissue. Adjuvant chemotherapy is mandatory.

➤ If the surgery is not too extensive, bone grafts might be attempted, but a better alternative is a metal or plastic prosthesis (artificial limb).

Brain

Brain tumors are serious and frightening—and often fatal. They occur most often in people over the age of 40 (85 percent) or under the age of 20 (15 percent). When a tumor is malignant, it can spread to other parts of the brain, and even if it does not spread, the tumor itself can expand and destroy healthy tissue. Brain tumors are classified according to the type of cell in which they arise, the most common being *astrocytoma, brain stem glioma,* and *ependymal tumor.*

➤ The tumor is removed, but as much normal tissue as possible is left intact in order to preserve neurologic function. Surgery, the type of which depends on the location and size of the tumor, is always followed by adjuvant chemotherapy and/or radiation.

Breast

Breast cancer is a general term for several different malignancies that arise in breast tissue, among them *ductal carcinoma, lobular carcinoma, Paget's disease of the nipple,* and *adenoid cystic carcinoma.* Breast cancer is very common but very treatable, and is second to lung cancer as the leading cause of cancer death in women.

➤ *Radical mastectomy,* done infrequently now, is removal of the entire breast, axillary lymph nodes, and the muscles under the breast. A modified radical mastectomy leaves the muscles intact.
➤ *Partial mastectomy* is removal of the entire tumor as well as a wide margin of breast tissue. This operation leaves a hole in the breast. The hole fills with lymph, which in time turns to soft scar tissue.
➤ *Lumpectomy* is removal of the tumor only, and is followed by radiation therapy.
➤ *Wide excision* is removal of the tumor with a wide margin of at least 1 cm.

➤ *Breast reconstruction* is now almost always done—by a plastic surgeon, at the time of the original cancer surgery. The two most commonly used techniques are *saline implant*, which is done in one stage for small-breasted women, and *tissue expansion*, which involves an inflatable *prosthesis* (artificial breast), which is inflated gradually in the doctor's office every few weeks after surgery. The expandable prosthesis can be permanent, or it can be exchanged for a plastic implant.

Cervix

The cervix is the neck of the uterus, which extends down into the upper part of the vagina. Cervical cancer is very common but highly curable if detected early by a Pap test. Women at the greatest risk for cervical cancer are those who began having intercourse at an early age; those who have had multiple sex partners, especially if those partners were uncircumcised men; those who have had more than five pregnancies; and those whose mothers took *diethylstilbesterol (DES)* while they were pregnant.

➤ *Radical hysterectomy*, done only for advanced disease, is removal of the entire uterus, including the cervix, the upper third of the vagina, and all the supporting ligaments.
➤ *Modified radical hysterectomy* leaves in some of the supporting ligaments, which contain nerves that control bladder function.
➤ *Total hysterectomy* removes only the uterus and cervix. It is done through either the abdomen or vagina.
➤ *Radical pelvic exenteration*, done for very far advanced disease or for recurrence of cancer, removes all the important structures in the pelvis, including the bladder and rectum. It has many complications and a significant mortality rate.
➤ *Trachelectomy*, done to preserve fertility, removes only the cervix, and the uterus is sewn to the vagina.
➤ *Conization* is excision of a cone-shaped piece of tissue from the cervix, done with either a scalpel or laser. It is performed to diagnose as well as to treat cancer.

Colon

The colon is the large intestine, also called the *bowel*. People at greatest risk of colon cancer are those over age 40, those who have a family history of colorectal cancer, those who have polyps, or those who have a history of ulcerative colitis. Surgery is followed by adjuvant chemotherapy.

> ➢ Even if there is no significant metastasis, the tumor is always removed, along with a significant portion of the colon and the entire lymph node drainage. If the tumor is fairly small, the two ends of the bowel can be *anastamosed* (reconnected to one another).
> ➢ When the tumor is on the left side (where the colon connects to the rectum), or if there is partial or complete bowel obstruction, a temporary colostomy is performed.
> ➢ Small tumors or precancerous polyps can be removed by local excision, often via *colonoscopy*.

Esophagus

The esophagus is the tube that carries food from the mouth and throat to the stomach. Esophageal cancer is rare compared with other cancers of the gastrointestinal tract, but it is one of the least curable and rapidly fatal cancers. Its major cause is smoking, and it is more common in men than women.

> ➢ *Radical surgery* consists of removing the entire esophagus as well as surrounding tissues and lymph nodes. If the tumor is in the lower portion of the esophagus, the top of the stomach has to be removed too.
> ➢ If the tumor has invaded the trachea, a new swallowing tube can be inserted inside the esophagus in a palliative procedure.

Gallbladder

The gallbladder is a sac beneath the liver that stores bile, a substance that breaks down fat. Cancer of the gallbladder is rare, but it is three times more common in women than men.

> ➢ Surgery holds out the only hope of cure for cancer of the gallbladder, which is removed along with the lymph nodes and a wedge of healthy liver. Whether or not the tumor is fully removed, the surgeon must create a drainage system for the bile; this is usually done by placing a tube that leads to the small intestine.

Head and Neck

Head and neck cancer is a term that covers a variety of types of the disease that occur in the head (excluding the brain) and neck, including the upper air passages, mouth, sinuses, lips, tongue, gums, cheek, and tonsils. Almost all are squamous cell carcinomas.

➤ Depending on where the tumor is, it is removed along with the appropriate lymph nodes. The surgery is preceded and/or followed by radiotherapy and chemotherapy.

➤ Reconstructive surgery may be done if the head and neck surgery is radical—and it often is.

Kidneys

Kidney cancer is rare and affects about twice as many men (most of whom are over age 65) as women. It is more common in urban, industrialized areas and in people who smoke.

➤ *Partial nephrectomy* (removal of the kidney) can be done in patients with only one kidney or with small tumors in both kidneys.

➤ If both kidneys have large tumors, they will be removed, and the patient will then require lifelong kidney dialysis.

Liver

Liver cancer (hepatocellular carcinoma) is a primary cancer of the liver rather than cancer that spreads to the liver from another primary site (metastatic liver cancer). Although primary liver cancer is relatively rare in the United States (most often seen in people who have cirrhosis of the liver), metastatic liver cancer is very common.

➤ If the entire tumor can be removed, surgery can cure liver cancer because the liver has two lobes, and life can be easily maintained with only one.

➤ If both lobes are involved, however, most of the liver can be removed in a complex procedure called a trisegmentectomy, which is dangerous and not easily survivable when the patient has poor liver function.

➤ If the cancer has not metastasized but the tumor is very large, if there are multiple tumors, or the tumor involves both lobes, a liver transplant can be considered.

Lungs

There are two major types of lung cancer: *small cell* (also called undifferentiated small cell and, formerly, oat cell carcinoma) and *non-small cell*. The latter is by far the most common, but the single greatest cause of both types of lung cancer is cigarette smoking, especially for smokers who are exposed to environmental carcinogens. The disease is rarely diagnosed in its early stages, which is why it is so difficult to treat successfully.

➤ The tumor and the lobe of the lung in which it is located (and sometimes the entire lung) must be removed. The removal is followed with adjuvant chemotherapy.

Ovaries

The ovaries are located on top and to the side of the uterus and are connected to that organ by the *fallopian tubes*. The ovaries produce a variety of female hormones and are responsible for maturing an *ovum* (egg) each month during a woman's childbearing years. Ovarian cancer increases in incidence after age 50, which coincides with the average age of menopause. Because it is asymptomatic until well advanced, it is usually difficult to treat.

➤ In early-stage cancer, one or both ovaries and adjacent lymph nodes are removed, and adjuvant chemotherapy is given.
➤ In advanced disease, as much of the tumor as possible is removed, as well as the uterus and surrounding lymph nodes. Surgery is always followed by adjuvant chemotherapy.

Pancreas

The pancreas is the long gland that lies behind the stomach and that is responsible for producing insulin to metabolize dietary carbohydrates. Although pancreatic cancer is not common (the incidence rises after age 60), it is the fifth leading cause of cancer death and is thus one of the more lethal forms of the disease.

➤ Surgical removal of the tumor, as well as a small margin of healthy pancreatic tissue, might be sufficient to cure the cancer.

➤ When the tumor is too large or has metastasized, surgery may be done to reduce its size (debulk) it, and adjuvant chemotherapy is given. This may improve survival and quality of life.

➤ Depending on the location of the tumor, radical surgery called *pancreaticoduodenal resection* may be curative if the tumor is highly localized, but diagnosing pancreatic cancer in this stage is unlikely.

➤ Surgery also can be done to bypass obstruction of the biliary (pertaining to the gallbladder and bile ducts) or gastrointestinal tract.

Penis

Cancer of the penis is very rare in the United States. It is more common in elderly men, blacks, and men who have not been circumcised.

➤ Total or partial *penectomy* is done with either a scalpel or laser. If adjacent lymph nodes are enlarged or cancerous, they are excised.

➤ *Mohs micrographic* surgery is very limited excision of only the visible tumor. Additional small fragments are examined under the microscope and removed until all malignant tissue has been excised.

Pituitary Gland

The pituitary gland is located in the center of the brain above the back of the nose. Its major function is secretion of various hormones. Most pituitary tumors are benign, but on rare occasions, they turn malignant.

➤ In malignant tumors, the entire pituitary must be removed because the gland is so small (about the size of a pea), either through the nose (transphenoidal hypophysectomy) or through the skull (craniotomy). Replacement hormones and other drugs are given after surgery.

Prostate Gland

The prostate gland, one of the male sex glands, is situated below the bladder and in front of the urethra. Prostate cancer is extremely common, but since the average age at diagnosis is 73, and because it is very slow growing, many men die of other causes before they know they have prostate cancer. In fact, many cases of prostate cancer are diagnosed only at autopsy. Prostate cancer is highly curable if diagnosed and treated early on.

- ➤ *Radical prostatectomy* is removal of the entire prostate gland, the seminal vesicles, nerves to the penis, and all pelvic lymph nodes. About 30 to 50 percent of men suffer postoperative impotence. This is the only surgical technique that has a chance of being curative.
- ➤ *Incomplete prostatectomy* removes the part of the prostate gland that becomes enlarged in benign prostatic hypertrophy (noncancerous enlargement of the prostate). There are a number of ways to perform the procedure, but none is used as a complete cure for the disease.
- ➤ *Cryosurgery* is used for both malignant disease and for benign prostatic hypertrophy.

Rectum

The rectum is the lowest four to six inches of the colon and is connected to the anus. Feces collect in the rectum, and when there is a sufficient mass, you feel the urge to defecate. Rectal cancer is fairly common, more so in men than women, and risk increases significantly over age 40. Those at greatest risk have a family history of colorectal cancer and/or a history of ulcerative colitis.

- ➤ A tumor with a 2 cm margin is removed, as are the regional lymph nodes. Preoperative radiation therapy is often given to shrink the size of the tumor. This results in the best chance of preserving the sphincter muscle, which allows you to control your bowels. However, if the tumor is very low in the rectum, the entire structure, as well as the anus, is removed, resulting in a permanent colostomy.

➤ If the tumor is very small, it can be removed by wedge resection (cutting out the tumor with surrounding normal tissue in the shape of a slice of pie) under local anesthesia.
➤ In noninvasive tumors, it is possible to do cryosurgery from below (through the anus).
➤ Local incision or ablation (removal of diseased tissue by scraping or by laser) is performed when the tumor is small and confined only to the rectum. In this procedure, the surgeon makes an attempt to leave the sphincter muscle intact, and over the course of four or five treatments, the tumor is removed by laser or fulguration.

Skin

There are two major types of skin cancer: basal cell carcinoma and malignant melanoma.

Basal Cell Carcinoma

Basal cell carcinoma accounts for more than 90 percent of all skin cancers and is highly curable. It is essentially a disease of people who are middle-aged or older and is a function of skin pigmentation (the fairer the skin, the greater the risk) and exposure to the sun.

➤ In *electrodessication and curettage*, the cancer is burned and scraped.
➤ *Cryosurgery* freezes the cancerous lesion.
➤ In *excision*, the entire cancerous lesion is removed along with a margin of normal tissue. This can be done with a scalpel or a laser.

Malignant Melanoma

Often called "the disease that gives cancer a bad name," malignant melanoma is a particularly virulent type of skin cancer most common in white people who have many moles. Success of treatment depends almost entirely on the stage at which it is diagnosed. If it is caught early, it is curable with surgery and adjuvant chemotherapy.

➤ Complete removal of the primary tumor with very wide margins is the treatment of choice, often followed by adjuvant chemotherapy. Adjacent lymph nodes also are excised even if they are not enlarged. The amount of healthy tissue removed depends on the size and depth of the tumor.

Small Bowel

The small bowel, also called the small intestine, extends from the bottom of the stomach to the point where it is joined by the large intestine. Cancer of the small bowel is much rarer than the disease in the large bowel. People who suffer from Crohn's disease are at particular risk.

➤ The tumor is removed, and depending on the extent of the metastasis, part of the liver also may be removed. This is followed by adjuvant chemotherapy.

Stomach

The incidence of stomach cancer has been declining dramatically in the United States, perhaps because of the decreasing use of nitrate-containing food preservatives. Compounds containing nitrogen have been causally associated with the disease. Almost all stomach cancers are adenocarcinomas, and there may be a hereditary risk factor.

➤ *Radical surgery* means that all or most of the stomach is removed along with surrounding lymph nodes. It is almost always followed by adjuvant chemotherapy. If the tumor is particularly invasive, part of the small intestine also is removed.

➤ If a cure is deemed impossible, *palliative surgery* is done to prevent fatal hemorrhage or to relieve obstruction.

Testes

The testes are the male reproductive glands. Testicular cancer is very rare and usually occurs in only one testicle. It is most common in men ages 20 to 24, especially those who have suffered from cryptorchidism: failure of the testes to descend.

➤ For localized tumors, the testis, epididymis, and spermatic cord are removed (*radical orchiectomy*). Lymph nodes may or may not be excised depending on the presence of metastasis. Although a man will be impotent following the surgery, fertility can be preserved by donating sperm before the operation.

Thyroid Gland

Thyroid cancer is rare and occurs much more frequently in women than men, particularly women of childbearing age. The greatest risk factor for thyroid cancer is a past history of radiation treatment for conditions such as tonsillitis, ear infection, ringworm of the scalp, or any other diseases of the head and neck. Radiation for these diseases was common prior to the widespread use of antibiotics to treat such infections. Thyroid cancer grows slowly and rarely metastasizes.

➤ When almost the entire thyroid gland is removed, the patient has the best chance of cure, especially when the cancer occurs in several places in the gland.

➤ When the cancer is small and confined to only one lobe of the gland, that is all that is removed (lobectomy).

Uterus

The *endometrium* is the lining of the uterus and fairly often gives rise to the most common type of cancer: adenocarcinoma. The risk of endometrial cancer rises after menopause and is higher in women who have a family history of the disease, women who have diabetes and/or who are obese, and women who have never been pregnant.

➤ The uterus, cervix, both fallopian tubes, both ovaries, and the pelvic lymph nodes are excised. This is followed by adjuvant chemotherapy.

Vagina

Vaginal cancer (squamous cell carcinoma) is rare and almost always occurs in women over age 50. An even rarer type of vaginal cancer, known as clear cell adenocarcinoma, is seen in young women and adolescents, particularly those whose mothers took DES while they were pregnant.

➤ *Radical vaginectomy* includes radical hysterectomy and the removal of all pelvic lymph nodes. Skin grafts are sometimes necessary, and narrowing of the vaginal canal is a common postoperative complication.

➤ *Conservative surgery* involves excision of only the vagina and pelvic lymph nodes.

Vulva

Cancer of the vulva is slightly more common than vaginal cancer, although still very rare, and it occurs almost exclusively after menopause. Women who have a history of *leukoplakia* (a white, thickened patch on the vulva) are at higher risk of vulvar cancer, and many physicians believe that leukoplakia is a precursor to cancer, in the same way that cervical polyps may be a precursor to cervical cancer.

➤ Radical vulvectomy means removing the entire vulva, as well as all the lymph nodes on both sides of the groin. Infection is a common complication because of breakdown of the incision. If this occurs, it takes months to heal, and there will most likely be significant scarring.

➤ Modified vulvectomy removes only half of the vulva and the lymph nodes only on the side where the tumor is located. Infection is less likely after this procedure, but there may be constant swelling of the leg on the side where lymph nodes were removed.

➤ Local excision removes only the tumor with a 2-cm margin. It is done with either a scalpel or laser. Pelvic lymph nodes are then removed by laparoscopy, a procedure in which a laparoscope, with fiberoptic light attached, is inserted through a small abdominal incision.

Chapter Nine

Pain

Cancer May Hurt, but Pain Can Be Controlled

*M*ore often than not, cancer—and its treatment—hurts.
There's no escaping this fact, but you *can* escape from,
or significantly minimize, the pain. Up until recently, oncologists
(and most other physicians and nurses as well) didn't give much
thought to pain control, either because they believed that pain is an
inevitable part of the disease, or because they were afraid of the
effects of long-term use of narcotic analgesics. And in some cases,
with some doctors, plain old insensitivity was at work.

Some feared investigation by state and regulatory agencies if
they prescribed adequate amounts of pain medication, narcotics
especially, on an effective dosing schedule. And again, up until
recently, there were no scientifically controlled studies of pain relief
to buck traditional patterns of medical practice that ignored or minimized chronic cancer pain.

Prior to the last decade or so, pain relief in hospitals and outpatient clinics was notoriously inadequate, and in some places it still is.
Partly as a result of the consumer movement in health care and
partly as a result of better and more realistic education of health care
providers, things have improved, and you don't have to put up with
outmoded and paternalistic beliefs and practices. Excellent pain relief
is available, and it is your right to receive it. If your complaints of
pain are not dealt with in a positive and sensitive way, you and your
family should insist—demand, if necessary—that your pain be
treated. After all, pain has no redeeming value. Physical suffering

doesn't teach you anything about life or about having cancer (except that it exists—and you already knew that), and it certainly doesn't build character.

In addition to the other patients and families who demand pain relief, and in addition to better education of health care personnel, you have a new powerful ally. In July 1999, The Joint Commission on the Accreditation of Healthcare Organizations (JCAHO) approved new standards of pain assessment and control. This is a major boon for cancer patients because the JCAHO accredits 80 percent of American hospitals (98 percent of all licensed beds—which includes yours) and is an extremely powerful organization. Hospitals are inspected for re-accreditation every three years, and the doctors, nurses, and administrators take a JCAHO accreditation inspection *very* seriously. In other words, if the JCAHO says to do something, hospitals hop to it. And beginning in 2001, the pain assessment and control standards will be part of the accreditation process. A synopsis of the standards follows:

- ➤ Recognition of patients' right to pain assessment
- ➤ Pain assessment for all patients, documentation of the assessment, and follow-up assessments
- ➤ Education about pain control for all appropriate hospital personnel and determination that they are competent to assess and control pain
- ➤ Institution of policies and procedures that support prescription of adequate pain medication
- ➤ Assurance that pain does not interfere with rehabilitation
- ➤ Patient and family education about pain management while in the hospital and as part of discharge planning
- ➤ Collection of hospital-wide data to measure effectiveness of pain management

Why Cancer Hurts

First, we need to define pain in general. That's easy, you may think. Pain is anything that hurts. This is true, but only from the point of view of the person experiencing the pain. No one else can feel your pain, but physicians can understand what it is because there are objective neurological parameters to discern and measure it.

Nerve endings called *nociceptors* react in the face of certain noxious stimuli that we call pain. These nociceptors receive the painful signals and send them along to the brain, which in effect says, "Ouch!"

In cancer, nociceptors receive noxious stimuli for a number of reasons:

> ➤ A tumor has invaded healthy tissue such as bones, blood vessels, and muscles.
> ➤ A tumor is exerting pressure on hollow organs and tubes such as the stomach, intestines, esophagus, and bile duct.
> ➤ A tumor is pinching nerves.
> ➤ A tumor is producing inflammation of a tissue or structure.
> ➤ A tumor is blocking blood vessels or lymph nodes, thus causing *edema* (swelling), which leads to pain.
> ➤ There are other complications of the cancer and/or its treatment, such as bowel or bladder obstruction, peptic ulcers, burning of the hands and feet, skin problems from radiation, and the like.

All this hurts to varying degrees.

One of the most serious and troubling sources of pain is when cancer either arises from or metastasizes to bones, usually those in the limbs, pelvis, and vertebrae. Many times, bone pain is *referred pain*—that is, it arises someplace else and is "referred" via neural pathways to the place where you experience it. For example, cancer that has metastasized to the spine might actually spread down one or both legs.

In addition to the strictly physical characteristics, other factors contribute to pain and may increase its severity:

> ➤ The longer the pain continues unrelieved, the greater your suffering and anxiety, which in turn leads to more pain—a true vicious circle.
> ➤ Pain makes you angry, which makes you tense and anxious—and more likely to feel pain.

➤ Unrelieved pain makes the general healing and recovery process take longer, which adds to the economic and psychological cost of cancer treatment.

➤ Pain strips you of dignity, and if it's bad enough, it interferes with every single aspect of your life. In the face of severe, agonizing pain, nothing else matters, and it's almost impossible to think about anything but the pain.

➤ Severe, agonizing cancer pain makes some people think that they don't want to go on living. This depression makes the pain worse. This is the worst possible scenario for cancer patients.

Everyone reacts somewhat differently to pain, and some people have higher pain thresholds than others, but there is no reason for you to be caught up in an escalating spiral of fear, pain, and anxiety. You can and will receive pain relief.

Painful Treatment

Sometimes the treatment for cancer hurts as much or more than the disease itself. It almost goes without saying that you're going to have pain following surgery, and it doesn't always go away when you would think the recovery period is over. Long-term painful effects of cancer surgery include:

➤ Tight, burning sensations or numbness or prickliness after radical neck dissection for head and neck cancer

➤ Constricting, burning pain in the back of the arm, the armpit, and in the chest (especially upon movement) after mastectomy

➤ Ache, extreme soreness, or loss of feeling along the scar after thoracotomy for lung cancer

➤ Numbness or heaviness in the side and front of the abdomen or in the groin after nephrectomy for kidney cancer

➤ Phantom pain or stump pain after amputation of a leg or arm for bone cancer

Chemotherapy can hurt too. Needle sticks are no fun, and even when a vascular access device is inserted (a catheter or port that is surgically placed under the skin, with a tube leading into a major vein), there is still a needle puncture, although not a venipuncture, every time you receive a dose of chemotherapy.

Some drugs cause pain as they are flowing into the vein. These are called *vesicants* and are extremely irritating to tissue. (Appendix A includes a list of these drugs.) Also during chemotherapy, some of the drug can leak out of the vein, a condition called *extravasation*, which can be slightly irritating or very painful. If you feel undue pain or burning during your infusion, tell the doctor or nurse so they can stop further tissue damage. Other drugs cause *peripheral neuropathy*, which causes tingling, numbness, or pain in the extremities because the drugs damage peripheral nerves. This is especially true with vincristine, vinblastine, cisplatin, and taxotere.

Myths and Misconceptions
Before we go further and discuss pain relief, you ought to be aware of some misconceptions about cancer and pain.

➤ Having cancer doesn't *necessarily* mean you will be in pain, and if you are, it may not be severe, and it surely won't be constant. The pain of cancer is not inevitable.

➤ If something does hurt, there is no reason to believe that it will inevitably get worse or that it will always be there. Sometimes the treatment itself, especially surgery, alleviates pain without analgesics.

➤ The pain does not mean that the cancer is incurable. That's what chemotherapy, as well as surgery and radiation, are for: to cure or palliate the disease so you will be disease free or in remission—and pain free.

➤ It is *not true* that analgesics, even potent narcotics, will negatively affect the progress of the disease or that you will become addicted to them. It is almost unheard of for a cancer patient, or anyone else in severe pain, to become addicted to medically prescribed narcotics. Addiction is usually a "voluntary" problem and the result of severe emotional illness.

➤ You will not walk around in a "drugged" state—or not be able to walk around at all—while you are taking analgesics, even narcotics. When the dose is adjusted properly and, after a few days, your system has gotten used to the medication, you should be able to function well.

➤ Many people think that moderate to severe pain can be relieved only by injections. Oral medications work very well if the dose is adequate and the dosing schedule is maintained. The key to making oral pain medication work effectively is to gradually raise the dose until pain is relieved—and then stick with that dose around the clock.

Assessing Pain

You are the only one who can feel your pain. In fact, unless you choose to tell people, you are the only one who knows you're in pain. Therefore, if you want to relieve it, you'll have to speak up. Some physicians and nurses will ask if you're having pain, especially if they see you wincing or screwing up your face, or exhibiting other signs of pain, but most probably will not. They will expect you to mention it and ask for help. So ask. There are several good reasons not to suffer in silence:

➤ The longer you wait, the worse the pain will get. The worse the pain is, the longer it will take the analgesic to kick in, and the bigger the dose you will need.

➤ It doesn't do you any good to keep a stiff upper lip. You're not going to score points for "bravery," and the only one you're hurting is yourself. No one will think the less of you for asking for relief.

➤ Pain, and its quality and intensity, is one of the ways your oncologist can measure the progress of the disease and the effects of the treatment. If your doctor doesn't know everything that's going on, he or she may be hampered in making decisions about chemotherapy.

➤ Pain may be a side effect of chemotherapy, and your oncologist needs to know this.

➤ Anxiety, fear, and worry can increase pain, and if you are unwilling to ask for pain relief, you'll only become more anxious, afraid, and worried—even if you don't know you are.

Describing the Pain

The minute you tell the doctor it hurts, he or she will ask questions. In order for you to achieve the best possible pain control, try to answer them as carefully and thoughtfully as you can. It's not that the doctor is testing you, it's that he or she needs to know what the pain feels like in order to prescribe the right drug at the right time. These are some of the things you'll be asked about:

> ➤ *How long the pain lasts.* Does it appear suddenly and ebb fairly quickly, or does it appear gradually, perhaps increasing in intensity, and hang around for a long time, sometimes months? If the former, you'll be diagnosed as having *acute pain*, which can arise from the tumor itself (removal almost always relieves the pain) or from the chemotherapy. The latter is characterized as *chronic pain*, which may ebb and flow in intensity but is always there.

> ➤ *Where the pain is located. Focal pain* emanates from a specific place, usually where the tumor is. Pain that seems to spread out over a wide area (which is actually along the length of a nerve) is called *radiating pain*. If the source of the pain is in an organ or a tissue that does not have pain receptors, other tissues along the same network send pain signals to the brain. This is called *referred pain*. The most common example of referred pain is right shoulder pain as a result of gallbladder disease. You'll also be asked if the pain moves around or stays in one place and whether it increases in intensity when you move around.

> ➤ *What type of pain it is.* This may be difficult for you to assess because all you really know is that it hurts. But physicians distinguish between types of pain. *Organic pain* is actual pain, and it is the usual source of cancer-related pain (as contrasted with *psychosomatic pain*, which originates in the mind—but is nevertheless very real). There are three types of organic pain: *somatic pain* affects pain receptors and causes dull achiness in a specific area; *visceral pain* is less focused and feels like squeezing and pressure, often accompanied by nausea, vomiting, and sweating; *neuropathic pain* arises from damage to nerves and feels like burning, stabbing, or being caught in a vise.

You also will be asked:
> ➤ To rate the intensity of the pain on a scale of 1 to 10, with 10 being the most severe

➤ To describe the pattern of the pain—that is, how it comes and goes, what makes it worse and what eases it
➤ Whether you have ever had pain like this before and what you've done to relieve it (and how well those measures worked)
➤ Whether it prevents you from sleeping
➤ Whether it affects your mood and appetite

You will probably be physically examined as an additional way to evaluate the nature and intensity of the pain.

If no one asks you about your current pain medication, be sure to volunteer the information. What drugs are you taking now, in what dose, and how often? How long does it take for the medication to work—or does it work at all? Do you have side effects, and are they so bad that you don't want to take the drug anymore? Good pain interviewers (physicians or nurses) also will make an assessment of your emotional state because it has such a profound effect on physical pain.

Controlling Pain

There are a number of ways to control pain. Using drugs is the most common method, and for most types of pain, it is effective. However, for intractable pain, a surgical, anesthetic, or radiological approach can be used, and some patients prefer nonmedical interventions such as hypnosis or acupuncture. In many cases, the cancer treatment itself (surgical, chemotherapeutic, or radiological) relieves pain because it shrinks the tumor and thus lessens pressure on surrounding organs, tissue, and nerves.

The important thing is not the method used to control pain but rather the consistency with which it is applied, as well as the faith that both you and your physician have in the method. An aggressive, consistent approach to pain relief is essential.

Pharmacologic Pain Relief

Most cancer pain can be relieved through *analgesics* (drugs that relieve pain) that do not produce loss of consciousness and that allow you, for the most part, to go about your daily activities.

The effectiveness of analgesic drugs depends on a variety of factors: the type and intensity of pain, the drug itself, and the way in which it is administered. The World Health Organization, out of concern for cancer patients who were not receiving effective pain relief, devised a "ladder" approach to pain management. This approach starts with the simplest and mildest drugs and proceeds up the ladder to the most powerful narcotic analgesics until the pain is controlled.

There is no such thing as the best pain medication or a "standard" dose. Pain is highly individual, as is pain relief, and a drug and dose that is sufficient to ease one person's cancer pain may be insufficient for another's. The best way to manage cancer pain is to *titrate* dosage—that is, to increase or decrease the amount of medication until pain is relieved. The goal is to take an adequate amount of medication (one or a combination of drugs) that best controls the pain and produces the fewest side effects.

> ➤ The first step is to use a nonnarcotic analgesic, such as aspirin, acetaminophen, and propoxyphene, or *nonsteroidal anti-inflammatory drugs (NSAID)*, such as ibuprofen, naproxen, and ketoprofen. They can be used alone or in combination with one another, or with adjuvant medications. Nonnarcotic analgesics act on the central nervous system by rendering it somewhat insensitive to the perception of pain. They won't make you drowsy or "happy" or unconsciousness, and they don't cause *tolerance* (the condition in which more and more of a drug is needed to achieve the same effect) or *dependence* (physical and/or psychological need for a drug). There is, however, a *ceiling dose*, a point beyond which more of the drug will not do any good. For instance, four aspirin will not be more effective in relieving a headache than two.

> ➤ The second step is a weak or mild *narcotic analgesic* (also called an *opioid*), such as codeine, hydrocodone, and oxycodone, given alone or in combination with the drugs used in Step 1. Weak narcotics given alone in low doses work only about as well as aspirin or acetaminophen; they are much more effective when used in combination. Weak narcotics are almost always given orally, but some are available as rectal suppositories (which work very quickly) if you have trouble swallowing.

➤ The third step is to use a potent opioid, such as morphine, methadone, oxymorphone, fentanyl, hydromorphone, levorphanol, and meperidine, given alone or in combination with NSAIDs or other drugs. None of these drugs is considered better than another, although morphine and hydromorphone are used most often. These opioids are given orally when they are used to treat chronic pain, but they work faster and more effectively for acute pain if administered intramuscularly or intravenously. Most also can be given as rectal suppositories. It is general practice to start with the lowest effective dose of a strong narcotic and gradually increase it until either the pain is relieved or until side effects become intolerable. In the face of chronic cancer pain, the best way to give these drugs is every four hours around the clock, with "rescue doses" for breakthrough pain. At first, this may seem excessive (why give a narcotic if you're not in pain at the moment), but keeping a certain level of narcotics in the bloodstream is the most effective way to maintain adequate pain control. It also means that you don't have to keep asking for pain medication, which can be embarrassing and awkward. A few narcotic analgesics, notably morphine and oxycodone, are available in a long-acting form and are used mostly for very severe pain. They should be taken orally, and the pill must be swallowed whole—no crushing or chewing. The medication is then released slowly over an 8- or 12-hour period.

Side Effects

As with chemotherapeutic agents, all analgesic agents have side effects, some more serious than others. As a general rule, the higher on the pain relief ladder you go, the greater the risk of side effects, and the more serious they can be.

Nonnarcotic analgesics are generally very safe, but aspirin can cause gastrointestinal (GI) bleeding, especially after prolonged use (buffered aspirin is available to prevent GI bleeding). It is *contraindicated* (should not be used) in people who are taking coumadin or other blood thinners or chemotherapeutic drugs that tend to cause bleeding. In addition, if you have been allergic to aspirin in the past, don't take it now, and if you have a history of ulcers, stay away from aspirin. In high doses or after prolonged use, aspirin also can cause tinnitis (ringing in the ears), hearing loss, rapid heart rate and respiration, nausea and vomiting, and diarrhea.

Acetaminophen, when taken as directed on the package, almost never causes side effects, and it does not have the potential for GI bleeding that aspirin does. But high doses of acetaminophen taken every day for a long period of time can cause liver or kidney damage.

NSAIDs also are extremely safe, and there are so many of them that if you do get side effects from one brand, it is easy to switch to another. Although these problems are very rare, watch out for interference with blood clotting (if you have a low platelet count, don't take them), nausea and vomiting, indigestion, constipation, dizziness, headache, tinnitis, fluid retention, and rapid heart beat.

Narcotics do have side effects, some of them serious and almost all of them dose- and route-related. That is, the higher the dose, the greater the likelihood of adverse events, and the more directly the drug enters the bloodstream, the faster the side effects will appear and the more significant they will be. In descending order of route of administration, the speed at which narcotics (and all other drugs as well) reach the bloodstream are: intravenous, rectal, intramuscular, and oral. Although less common, especially for pain medication, drugs can be administered sublingually (a tablet placed under the tongue and allowed to dissolve), subcutaneously (injected just under the skin), epidurally (placed into a space along the spinal cord), transnasally (sprayed or dropped into the nose), or transdermally (via a skin patch).

The most common untoward reaction of narcotic analgesics is constipation. In fact, virtually no one receiving regular doses of morphine or other opioid drugs avoids constipation. Circumvent this by drinking lots of water, eating extra dietary fiber, or taking stool softeners or laxatives before it becomes a serious problem.

The other very common side effect is drowsiness, lethargy, and the feeling that your thinking ability is not functioning at peak form. (This could actually benefit you if you have been having trouble sleeping because of pain, anxiety, or depression.) Other people find themselves nauseated, which can be relieved by antiemetics.

Respiratory depression (slow, shallow breathing) can occur with high doses of morphine given for short periods of time for acute pain. It doesn't usually happen with lower doses over long periods, although it's something to be on the lookout for. Other uncommon side effects of narcotics include muscle twitching, dry mouth, urinary retention, and itching.

Fear of Addiction

We should say another word here about the fear of addiction to narcotics, because the belief that cancer patients turn into drug addicts is so commonplace. *It is simply not true.* People who take narcotics to relieve cancer pain, even for long periods of time—even for the rest of their lives—are not at risk of becoming addicted to the drugs. Unfortunately this myth is almost as widespread in the health care community as it is among the general public, and it is one of the major reasons why cancer patients have traditionally been so undermedicated for pain, as well as why so many cancer patients have been reluctant to talk about the true extent of their pain and ask for relief.

Drug addiction is a disease in and of itself—a mental illness—and it has nothing to do with having cancer. It is based on two physical and psychological factors: tolerance and dependency. Tolerance means that more and more of a drug is needed to achieve the same effect, and it rarely happens to cancer patients unless the pain itself is increasing in severity—and then it's a function of the amount of pain, not the drug or your reaction to it. If this happens (and it does *not* mean that you are becoming addicted), the appropriate response is to increase the dose or frequency of administration or switch to another drug.

Dependence is another story. Requiring a drug to alleviate actual physical pain is *not* the same as being dependent on that drug as a drug addict is dependent on his or her regular "fix." There are two types of drug dependence: physical and psychological. After you have taken narcotics for a certain amount of time (which varies from individual to individual), physical dependence is a normal and predictable consequence. It is not particularly problematic. If you stop taking the narcotics suddenly, you will have withdrawal symptoms: sweating, shaking, chills, and anxiety. Also, the pain will get worse. However, if you stop taking the narcotics gradually by reducing the dose and lengthening the time interval between doses, nothing happens. It is important to remember that *physical dependence is not the same as addiction.*

Psychological dependence, however, is a different matter. This is what is known as addiction. Since you are not a drug addict, we won't spend much time on the issue. Suffice it to say, though, that psychological dependence is a need to satisfy emotional, social, and psychological problems with drugs—not to solve a medical problem. One thing has nothing to do with another, and there is no reason for you to worry about being a drug addict, regardless of how long you take narcotics for physical pain.

Adjuvant Drugs
Other drugs can be used along with narcotic and nonnarcotic analgesics to help relieve pain. They are called *adjuvant drugs* and often have a potentiating effect (an effect that is greater than the sum of the two drugs).

Tricyclic antidepressants such as amitryptyline, doxepin, imipramine, and others, given at doses lower than that used for treating depression, help relieve the burning pain caused by cancer cell infiltration of nerves. Anticonvulsants such as carbamazepine relieve sharp or stabbing pains caused by tumors that press on nerves. They also are effective in postoperative pain and for stump pain after limb amputation. Corticosteroids such as dexamethasone and prednisone are very helpful in treating back pain due to spinal cord compression, metastasis to the bone, and nerve infiltration of cancer cells. Corticosteroids often improve appetite and mood and may have a positive effect on certain types of tumors. People who take them usually require less narcotic analgesia.

Surgical Pain Relief
When analgesics, even high doses of narcotics, don't work, surgery in the form of *neuroablation* is available. Neuroablation cuts or destroys (with a scalpel or, more often, with an electric cautery) pain fibers and thus interrupts the pathway that sends pain signals to the brain. This is highly sophisticated surgery and should be performed only by a neurosurgeon experienced in pain control. Also, it's not for everyone. Neuroablation is effective only on highly localized pain, and there are some serious potential side effects, the scariest of which is temporary or permanent loss of motor control (the ability to move voluntary muscles) in the part of the body that was operated on.

A *nerve block* uses a local anesthetic, which may be combined with cortisone, injected into or around a nerve to numb or deaden the fibers. It provides temporary pain relief, which is all that may be required. For more long-lasting relief, phenol (a strong antiseptic) can be injected. The downside of a nerve block is that it may deaden all sensory nerves in the area, which makes one vulnerable to serious injury. For instance, if it doesn't hurt when you stub your toe, you may not know you've broken it.

Cordotomy is a surgical procedure that interrupts the transmission of pain signals to the brain by cutting bundles of nerves in the spinal cord. It can be done either through an open incision in the back or through the skin (called *stereotactic surgery*). The major disadvantage of cordotomy is that sometimes other nerves are severed, such as those that transmit pressure or temperature. Cordotomy is highly effective in relieving pain for about three months or so, after which efficacy drops significantly.

Anesthetic Nerve Blocks and Stimulants

Various local anesthetics can be injected into or around nerve tissue to achieve temporary pain relief. This method works well only if a tumor has invaded tissue that can be fairly easily reached and that causes well-defined local pain. More than one nerve, or even several nerves, may have to be blocked in order to relieve pain, and the more extensive the block, the greater the potential for side effects, which can include urinary or rectal incontinence, motor weakness or loss of some motor control, and tingling and burning sensations (*paresthesia*).

In advanced metastatic disease involving the pelvis or lower body when pain cannot be well controlled with analgesics, *continuous epidural infusion* can be effective. A small reservoir is surgically implanted in the body with a thin catheter running into the spinal canal. An infusion pump delivers small doses over time so that the effect is a continuous level of analgesia.

Although it might seem counterintuitive, stimulating nerves can relieve pain. The trick is to send signals that are gentle rather than painful (for example brisk rubbing, pressure, or temperature changes), thus overriding the painful stimuli and preventing them from reaching the brain. It works well but only for a short time. *Transcutaneous electrical nerve stimulation (TENS)* is a technique in which an electrical device is placed over a painful area to stimulate the nerves. It works only when current is actually flowing and then only for a few months. It is also possible to implant a small variation of a TENS device.

Nonmedical Pain Relief

Acupuncture and acupressure have been used successfully for many centuries to relieve pain, and it works well for many people. Refer to Chapter 11 for a description of what acupuncture is and how it works.

Other nonmedical pain relief techniques may work for a while. They are usually most effective for people who have intermittent predictable pain that is associated with certain things, such as a treatment or procedure; incidental pain that flares up occasionally; and chronic pain exacerbated by stress and anxiety. These techniques include:

> *Guided imagery*, in which you are instructed to close your eyes and imagine a situation in which you are rid of your pain
> *Hypnosis*, in which you are put into a trance and given a post-hypnotic suggestion that your pain will be relieved
> Various *relaxation techniques*, in which you learn to breathe deeply to relax muscles and reduce tension
> *Massage*, with or without vibration, which should be done only by a trained massage therapist, and which is beneficial in that the caring touch is often as comforting as the muscle stimulation
> *Prayer*, which is helpful for some people
> *Humor therapy*, which can be effective if the pain isn't bad enough to preclude seeing the absurd and ridiculous
> *Listening to music*, which works best if the pain isn't so bad that you can't concentrate on the music
> *Distraction*, which means concentrating on something that will take your mind off the pain (a movie in the VCR, a terrific book, an absorbing television program, a telephone conversation with someone interesting), and which works best after you have taken a dose of pain medication and are waiting for the full effect to kick in

➤ *Biofeedback,* in which sensing devices are used to monitor involuntary functions such as heart rate, blood pressure, and muscle tension and which register the decrease in these functions as you teach yourself to relax

➤ *Moderate exercise,* such as brisk walking or easy bicycle riding, which can tone muscles, provide distraction, increase energy, overcome fatigue, and decrease nausea and vomiting

➤ *Playing with and caring for a pet,* which greatly reduces stress, increases a sense of well being, and provides a loving and friendly creature who will listen to your troubles, soak up tears, and give licks and kisses whenever you need them

Chapter Ten

Nutrition and Chemotherapy

Providing Energy and Comfort by Eating Well

*B*ecause many chemotherapeutic drugs have a profound effect on the gastrointestinal system, there will be times when eating will be the furthest thing from your mind. The very thought of food may make you queasy, your mouth may hurt, and even driving by a pizza parlor may induce nausea. Moreover, the drugs may change your sense of taste and cause diarrhea and/or constipation, neither of which is an appetite enhancer. It's safe to say that everyone who undergoes chemotherapy experiences some nutritional deficits regardless of the type and severity of side effects.

Nevertheless, you have to eat. Chemotherapy itself depletes your strength and can even cause temporary malnutrition, so you don't want to compound the problem by denying yourself a balanced diet. Also, it's much easier—and better for you—to maintain adequate nutrition right from the start of chemotherapy than to have to fight your way back from being malnourished.

In addition to the drug's side effects and the way they make you feel, sometimes a drug's chemistry, in and of itself, can affect the body's ability to absorb nutrients. And if you are hospitalized, you face another problem: hospital food. Even if you feel like eating, the quality and preparation of the food may turn you right off—it does most people. And since you can't live on intravenous fluids and yogurt, you will need to depend on friends and family to bring in food that is appetizing and palatable.

Basic Nutrition

Food is one of the major things that affects normal health as well as the body's ability to recover from serious illness. All foods are made up of nutrients: carbohydrates, proteins, and fats, as well as vitamins and minerals. Each type of nutrient has its own effect on body tissue. The consequence of eating these nutrients depends on the total amount in your diet and on your own individual metabolism, which may be drastically affected by chemotherapy.

Carbohydrates

Carbohydrates, which are composed of a variety of sugar molecules, are known as sugars and starches and are the body's major source of energy. In addition, carbohydrates build and repair tissues and regulate most body functions. Without them, you would die. There are two major types: simple and complex. *Simple carbohydrates* are sugars such as lactose found in milk, glucose (also called dextrose), fructose (found in fruits and vegetables), and sucrose (cane or beet sugar).

Complex carbohydrates, so named because they are chemically more complicated than simple sugars, are found in starches such as bread, pasta, and rice, and some vegetables such as beans, potatoes, and corn. Fiber is a complex carbohydrate as well.

Both simple and complex carbohydrates are broken down by the body into glucose, which is one of the substances measured as a chemical component of blood. (Abnormally high blood glucose is known as *diabetes*, and abnormally low blood glucose is known as *hypoglycemia*.) Simple and complex carbohydrates are broken down at the same rate, and they both provide four calories per gram. However, different foods produce differing amounts of glucose, and two major factors influence the amount of glucose in your bloodstream: the amount of carbohydrates you eat at a meal and the speed with which the carbohydrate is converted into glucose. The latter depends on how big the servings of food are, whether it is cooked (cooked food is digested faster than raw), and how much liquid the food contains (the more liquid, the faster it is digested). In addition, if you eat carbohydrates in combination with other nutrients, the carbohydrates are digested more slowly.

Fiber

Fiber is a carbohydrate found in vegetables, grains, fruits, and nuts. It is the part of the plant that cannot be digested. Since it is not absorbed, it does not provide calories, but because it is so bulky, it helps make you feel full. Obviously, then, fiber is a good thing to eat when you're trying to lose weight. The only problem is that it's not particularly emotionally satisfying. (No one's mother ever said, "I'll give you a nice piece of broccoli if you behave yourself.")

Water-insoluble fiber, such as wheat bran, helps the digestive tract by keeping waste products moving through the intestines, thus preventing constipation. Water-soluble fiber (oat bran, wheat germ, legumes) slows the passage of food from the stomach into the intestines, and it may help lower cholesterol.

Proteins

Protein is the basic building material of human life; it is used to create and repair tissue. Much important body tissue is composed of protein: muscles, bones, organs, and chemicals such as hormones and neurotransmitters. Proteins also can provide energy in the absence of carbohydrates. For example, if you were to lose so much weight that you used up all your fat reserves and were not taking in enough carbohydrates to provide energy, your body would start breaking down muscles and other tissues to use the protein they contain to keep you going. This is one of the things that happens to people with anorexia nervosa—and one of the things you want to guard against while you are undergoing cancer treatment.

Twenty-two *amino acids*, combining with one another in an almost infinite number of sequences, form the basis of protein. Your body manufactures only 13 of the 22; therefore, the other 9 must come from the food you eat. Protein is found in both plant sources (grains, legumes, nuts) and animal sources (meat, poultry, dairy products, fish). Protein provides four calories per gram.

Fat and Cholesterol

Fat, even more than sugar, is what makes things taste good. You never hear people say that they would rather eat low-fat cheese or salad dressing instead of the regular kind. Fat molecules carry the flavor of foods, and when their globular little selves are removed from ice cream or cheese or cookies, much of the flavor is removed also.

Most people know that there is a difference between *saturated* and *unsaturated* fat. The former is generally solid at room temperature and comes from animal products (milk, eggs, meat), except for palm oil and coconut oil, which come from plants but are saturated. Unsaturated fat is a vegetable product (olive oil, corn oil, safflower oil) and is liquid at room temperature.

Cholesterol, which is not a fat but works in conjunction with fat in your body, is a waxy substance that gets into your bloodstream via two major routes: it is manufactured normally by your liver and intestines, or it enters through the food you eat. Fatty red meat, whole-milk dairy products, and eggs are examples of foods high in cholesterol.

Cholesterol is deposited on the walls of your arteries, where it builds up over the years, gradually narrowing the lumen (inside passage) of these blood vessels, limiting the amount of blood that can get through. Eventually, the artery may become completely clogged, resulting in a heart attack or stroke.

Your body manufactures two types of cholesterol: *high-density lipoprotein (HDL)* and *low-density lipoprotein (LDL)*. HDL is often called "good" cholesterol because one of its actions is to remove cholesterol from the arteries and carry it back to the liver, where it is reprocessed and sent on its way to be eliminated. LDL is deposited into the arteries, and is the kind of cholesterol you want to minimize in your diet.

Fats work in concert with cholesterol in the following ways. Saturated fat raises the level of LDL, which increases your chances of clogged arteries. Unsaturated fat is believed to lower LDL levels and may even help raise HDL. For this reason, you should make an effort to eat more polyunsaturated than saturated fats. Try not to eat more than 300 mg of cholesterol each day.

Vitamins and Minerals

Vitamins and *minerals* are an integral part of the nutritive value of food, and if you eat a balanced diet, you do not need to take additional vitamins in the form of pills. Taking *megavitamins* (huge doses of selected vitamins) has been touted as a cure-all for a number of ailments, including cancer, but megavitamins can be extremely harmful, and in some cases, fatal. The same holds true for minerals such as calcium, potassium, iron, and zinc. Some types of chemotherapy interfere with absorption of certain nutrients, especially the B vitamins, so your oncologist may recommend supplements.

You may have heard that certain vitamins—C, E, and beta-carotene, which is converted to Vitamin A in the body—are antioxidants and play a role in reducing the risk of cancer because they prevent the destruction of certain cells. This may or may not be true, but you can get a sufficient amount of these vitamins in a well-balanced diet, especially in foods with strong colors. Yellow and orange foods (carrots, sweet potatoes, cantaloupe) are rich in beta-carotene; dark green vegetables (broccoli, green peppers) contain lots of Vitamin C, and green, leafy vegetables (spinach, escarole) and whole-grain foods (cereal, breads) are a good source of vitamin E.

What to Eat Every Day

The U.S. Department of Agriculture has established recommendations for a well-balanced diet that will provide adequate nutrition from a wide variety of foods. Here's what you should be eating every day:

> ➤ Breads, cereals, and grains, including rice and pasta: 6 servings
> ➤ Vegetables, including dark-green, leafy vegetables; dry peas or beans; and potatoes: 3 or more servings
> ➤ Fruits: 2 or more servings
> ➤ Cooked, lean meat, poultry, or fish: 2 servings
> ➤ Milk products, including skim milk, yogurt, or cheese: 2 servings

If you want to eat candy, sweets, and desserts, do so sparingly.

Additional Nutritional Requirements

Depending on the drugs you are taking, and the extent to which they deplete your body of nutrients, you may need to consume up to 20 percent more nutrients than you did before you started chemotherapy. Here's why:

> ➤ The stress of having cancer and undergoing treatment can cause your body to burn huge amounts of energy, which you must replace.

➤ Cancer cells grow rapidly and consume many of the nutrients that would otherwise be available to normal cells. Again, you must replace them.

➤ Cancer cells may release chemicals into the bloodstream that speed the consumption of nutrients, and they may be one of the contributory factors in loss of appetite.

➤ Stress, worry, depression, and other psychological factors may speed metabolism and cause you to burn energy faster than normal.

Maintaining good nutrition will give you more strength than you'll have if your eating habits are poor. It also will make you resist some of the side effects of chemotherapy, and those to which you fall victim can be less severe and last for a shorter period of time. Adequate nutrition can keep your immune system functioning well, and it can provide a measure of protection against infection. You will feel better too.

There is some belief that a well-nourished body means well-nourished cancer cells. This sounds like a negative effect, but cells that are well-fed and well-oxygenated reproduce themselves more rapidly and efficiently, which means they are more susceptible to cytotoxic drugs. And if you are well-nourished, you are more able to withstand the rigors of high-dose chemotherapy.

Nutrition is extremely important in the natural healing process, so if you have had surgery or radiation that destroys normal tissue, eating well will help you recover more quickly. Try some of the following to add extra nutrients to your diet:

➤ Add powdered milk to recipes that can tolerate it: meatloaf or meatballs, cakes, pudding, casseroles, and anything with a milk or cream base, such as soup. Fortify skim or low-fat milk (2 percent) by adding powdered milk to it. It won't change the taste and it will double the protein.

➤ Eat regular ice cream instead of frozen yogurt, and don't eat sugar-free foods. Blend a scoop of ice cream into a glass of milk for extra calories.

➤ Drink a glass of commercial food supplement between meals for extra nutrients. It tastes better if it's chilled.

➤ Add raisins or dried figs, apples, and pears to your cereal. If you make hot cereal, cook it with oat bran added and use cream instead of milk on top.

Emotional Aspects of Eating

Most people take pleasure in food itself, in the rituals around preparing and serving it, and in the enjoyment of sharing it with others. While you are undergoing chemotherapy, some of those pleasures fly out the window, and sometimes it becomes a major effort to get down a bowl of cereal and milk. There are a number of factors in the psychological aspects of nutrition and chemotherapy.

If you don't feel like eating at all or are unable to finish a meal, this can have a tremendous effect on your family life and social life. If you have to rely on hospital food, you're probably not going to eat much. Your appetite will vary tremendously, and you may not know when you'll feel like eating and when you won't; this too will have a strong effect on your life. The vagaries of the drugs' side effects, which wax and wane during the course of treatment, will affect your appetite and ultimately your nutrition. You may lose (or sometimes gain) enough weight so your clothes don't look right or don't fit. And dealing with well-meaning friends and family who try to force you to eat, prepare things that you don't want to or can't eat, and become almost obsessed with *your* eating habits can become annoying.

People also will recommend "anti-cancer" diets to you. They mean well, but they don't realize that "medical" information in a supermarket tabloid or even a more reputable publication is not to be taken as fact—or as a prescription.

In the past decade or so, there has been an enormous amount written in the popular press about "cancer diets" and about foods that prevent cancer. There is some scientific evidence regarding particular nutrients that tend to *reduce the risk* of cancer, but that is a far cry from curing cancer with food or going on an anti-cancer diet.

Your best, and safest, bet is to stick with a well-balanced diet in which you can pack the most calories, carbohydrates, and protein into the smallest amount of food. This may be one of the only times in your life where you will count calories in the opposite direction— to see how many you can manage to consume. Calories are what your body burns as energy, and since chemotherapy requires so much energy, you should try to double your usual calorie intake. Here are some more things you can try:

➤ When you're at the grocery store, buy homogenized milk; regular (not low-fat) cheese, cottage cheese, and yogurt; and regular ice cream, not low-fat ice cream or frozen yogurt.
➤ Don't use reduced or low-calorie mayonnaise and salad dressing or low-sugar jams and jellies.
➤ If you like fish and poultry go ahead and eat them, but don't give up beef, pork, and lamb because you think they're too fatty.
➤ Leave some visible fat on the meat and the skin on the poultry before cooking.
➤ Use regular margarine or butter instead of low-fat, and put extra sugar on your food if you like things sweet.
➤ Eat dessert as often as you want.
➤ Make high-calorie cold drinks in the blender or food processor: ice cream, extra cream if you like it, fruit, an egg, maybe a little wheat germ. This makes a wonderful breakfast or snack.
➤ Eat things that take up little space in your stomach but provide a lot of calories and protein: cheese omelets, grilled cheese sandwiches, cottage cheese and sour cream (slice in some radishes or scallions for crunch). Cream soups serve the same purpose.

Weight Loss

Not everyone loses weight during chemotherapy, and some people even put on flesh. But weight loss is more common than weight gain. The major reason is that cancer cells rob energy from normal cells, and you don't feel well enough to eat enough to make up for this theft—so you get thinner.

Cancer patients who don't lose too much weight generally do better than people who do. It's not clear why this should be so, but serious weight loss may be one of the signs of the most aggressive types of cancer.

It's tempting to think, "Well, I needed to shed a few pounds anyway," but this is *not* the way to go on a diet. Furthermore, weight maintenance is an indication that you are able to tolerate the chemotherapy. If you lose too much weight, you may need to switch drugs or stop chemotherapy altogether. Also, sudden and drastic weight loss leads to weakness and anemia; in addition to using up stored fat, the body is losing skeletal muscle as well, and red blood cells are diminished.

How to Maintain Appetite and Good Nutrition

Because certain drugs deplete the body of specific nutrients, you might want to consult a nutritionist experienced in devising nutritional programs for chemotherapy patients. These specialists address specific nutritional needs, food preferences, and the state of your appetite. Most hospital nutritionists can help you with this.

Appetite Stimulation

You've been eating all your life and perhaps cooking for a good part of it, so you know best what you find appealing and what you don't. Being on chemotherapy may change that for a while, and your favorite foods may suddenly turn you off. In fact, most food may turn you off for a few days after treatment—or after surgery. As you progress through your course of chemotherapy, you'll learn to cope with the vagaries of your fluctuating appetite, but you might try some of these suggestions:

➤ Eat only foods you like.
➤ Eat in restaurants (or order takeout meals) so you don't have to deal with food preparation and cleanup.
➤ Have family members do the cooking and cleanup.
➤ Set the table nicely, use your best dishes, light a candle, eat on the patio in nice weather—whatever improves the aura of food consumption.
➤ If you have been spending a lot of time in bed or sacked out on the couch, try to sit at the table for meals. Get dressed—even if it's only jeans and a sweatshirt—and comb your hair.

➤ Eat with others as often as you can because it stimulates appetite in two ways: it engages you in conversation so you don't concentrate on not wanting to eat, and it encourages you to follow the example of others.

➤ Make the food on the plate look as attractive and appealing as possible.

➤ Spend time outdoors in fresh air, which stimulates the appetite.

➤ Exercise moderately, which accomplishes the same goal.

➤ Eat small meals frequently instead of large ones at "regular" mealtimes. Become a grazer. Eat off smaller dishes (use a salad plate instead of a dinner plate) and use smaller utensils (a salad fork for your entrée or a teaspoon for your soup). Fooling your eyes often fools your stomach.

➤ Serve yourself small portions at mealtimes.

➤ Snack frequently and always have food with you when you're away from home.

➤ Take advantage of feeling well by having something to eat. Make the most of breakfast because you're least likely to feel nauseated in the morning.

➤ Even when you're really hungry and feel great, don't gorge yourself. Keep the portions small and frequent.

➤ No matter how you feel, keep drinking liquids. Even if you think it'll come right back up, take teeny sips of tepid water. You do *not* want to become dehydrated and end up having to live on intravenous fluids and liquid nutrition through a tube in your nose.

➤ Brush your teeth or swish some mouthwash before you eat so your mouth feels clean and fresh.

If some foods no longer taste good to you, don't eat them. Eat only what you find appetizing. Try not to cook in metal pots and pans. You may be extremely sensitive to the faint metallic taste.

You might try having someone else do the cooking so you're not tired of the food before you begin to eat. Also, try highly textured foods that are crispy, crunchy, and chewy. Nutritional supplements almost always taste better very cold or shaken up in a blender or food processor—with some fruit added.

Combating Nausea

Chapter 7 goes into great detail about combating nausea, but while we're on the subject of food, we need to talk about eating even though you feel nauseated a good deal of the time. Here are some techniques that can help:

➤ Try to avoid having an empty stomach at any time. Eat something light and bland, such as crackers, rice, yogurt, plain skinless chicken, and so forth. Then if you do vomit, it's not nearly as bad as when you have an empty stomach. Dry heaves are particularly unpleasant.

➤ Eat small amounts of food frequently, and don't drink liquids with solid food. They make you feel fuller and more bloated. Emulate a cat, which eats only until it's satisfied and then goes back for a little more when it's hungry again. (A dog will wolf down anything and everything and then throw up on the rug!)

➤ If you are really nauseated and know that any food will come right back up, wait until you feel better. Sometimes you don't know you're going to vomit, but if it's inevitable, wait till the feeling passes. Vomiting will only worsen nutritional problems. After the nausea attack is over, start with small sips of tepid water, increase the amounts and frequency of clear liquids (such as broth, tea, apple juice, and flavored gelatin), and progress to a small, bland meal. Don't eat sweet foods when you feel nauseated or have been vomiting.

➤ Don't drink sugar-free soda and other beverages, and do use sugar instead of sugar substitutes in your coffee or tea. Sugar slows peristalsis (the wavelike movements of your gastrointestinal tract) and thus combats nausea.

➤ While you are nauseated, breathe slowly and deeply with your mouth open a little, and concentrate on the rhythm of your breathing. Or try relaxation techniques or activities that distract you from the nausea.

➤ Don't lie down flat for at least two hours after eating. Sit up or recline on the sofa or in a recliner chair with your head propped up.

Sore Mouth and Throat

If your mouth and throat hurt, try the following:

➤ Avoid crispy, crunchy, and dry foods. Instead, eat things that are moist, smooth, and easily mixed with saliva.

➤ Stimulate saliva production by sucking on hard candy, eating Popsicles, chewing gum, and the like. If your saliva is thick and sticky, rinse your mouth with warm water before eating. Drinking hot beverages also will help.

➤ If your mouth is very dry, drink fluids almost constantly. You'll feel the urge to anyway. Carry a water bottle with you when you go out.

➤ Try drinking chilled liquid commercial food supplements. They're cool, smooth, and nutritious.

➤ Stay away from hot, spicy foods like chili and salsa, and stick to cool, smooth foods while your mouth is sore. Let hot foods cool off before putting them in your mouth.

➤ If your mouth really hurts, puree food in a blender or food processor. You might even want to try baby food for a while. Liquid supplements are a good choice because they're bland and highly nutritious.

➤ Don't smoke or drink alcohol.

Special Problems Related to Radiation Therapy

If you are getting radiotherapy, you may have added problems with mouth and throat complications because radiation has a strong effect on rapidly growing tissue, which includes mucous membranes in the mouth, nose, throat, esophagus, small intestine, and rectum. These tissues usually heal a few weeks after radiation treatment is over, but while you are receiving the therapy, you may have the following problems:

➤ *Radiation mucositis*, especially as a result of treatment to the head and neck. Membranes lining the mouth and throat will become inflamed, and salty, spicy, or sharp-edged foods will hurt. This means stay away from pretzels, potato chips, salsa, chili, and similar foods. You also should stop smoking (and chewing tobacco) and drinking alcohol because these substances irritate the mouth. If the irritation and inflammation is so severe that you don't want to eat at all, try using a topical anesthetic such as viscous Xylocaine before meals.

➤ Dry mouth (*xerostomia*) occurs as a result of radiotherapy to the head and neck because the salivary glands are affected by radiation. This is almost always temporary unless the doses of radiation are very high, in which case you might have some degree of dry mouth for the rest of your life. There are a number of different brands of artificial saliva and moisturizing gels on the market that will help you eat. Also, increase your intake of fluids, and make liberal use of sauces and gravies to help soften dry, hard foods.

➤ Radiation can affect taste buds, and coupled with the thickening of saliva that sometimes occurs, it probably will make food taste like nothing at all. Most of the things you would ordinarily try to enhance the flavor of food will be irritating or painful to your mouth and throat. This condition disappears after the therapy, but there's not much you can do about it while treatment is taking place.

➤ *Radiation enteritis* affects the small intestine and rectum as a result of radiation to the abdomen and/or pelvis. Severity of symptoms correlates with the radiation dose and frequency of treatment, but it usually disappears after the course of treatment. Symptoms include nausea and vomiting (treatment of upper abdomen or stomach) and frequent bowel movements and/or watery diarrhea (treatment of pelvis or lower abdomen). Even if you never get radiation enteritis, follow all the recommendations in Chapter 7 for preventing and treating diarrhea. Also, concentrate on eating meat, fish, and poultry (but don't fry it); bananas, apples, and apple juice; white bread and toast; macaroni and other noodles; potatoes (not French fries); cooked mild vegetables such as asparagus, green beans, carrots, and squash; and processed foods such as cheese, peanut butter, buttermilk, and yogurt. If symptoms appear, you will need to take medication such as Kaopectate, Lomotil, Imodium, Donnatol, Paragoric, or Compazine.

Taste Changes

Your sense of taste never changes for the better while you're going through chemotherapy, but there are a few things you can do to get the bad taste out of your mouth and to avoid the unpalatable taste of some foods:

> Suck on hard candies such as lemon or peppermint drops during chemotherapy infusions if you find that the drugs produce a bitter taste sensation.

> When you're cooking, use more salt and seasonings. Go easy at first and then step up the amount you use in recipes.

> Meat often tastes metallic during chemotherapy. You may have to switch to chicken or fish for the duration, but before you give up meat, try marinating it first in an olive oil–based marinade, and don't cook the meat in metal pans.

> The taste of cool or cold foods doesn't change as much as warm or hot ones. Eat fewer hot foods and try sandwiches, cold vegetable salads, tuna fish, cold soups, and the like.

> Brush your teeth frequently and use mouthwashes that don't contain alcohol, which tends to dry mucous membranes.

Lactose Intolerance

Lactose intolerance as a result of some cancer drugs is temporary, but if you drink milk or eat most milk products while you are on those drugs, you'll have diarrhea—which you certainly don't need. Nonfat yogurt and regular buttermilk are easily tolerated because the lactase in milk has been changed during processing. Here are some other suggestions:

> Try soy milk in cooking, although it's not very pleasant to drink straight (unless you can find some that's flavored with chocolate or strawberry). Look in the dairy case for lactose-free milk and other dairy products.

> Read the label on prepared foods to see if they contain lactose.

Fatigue

As we have already discussed, fatigue is one of the most common side effects of cancer and chemotherapy, and in some ways it's harder to cope with than pain or other problems because there's no pill to take to make it go away.

Fatigue and lack of appetite play off one another . You're too tired to cook, or even to eat what others have prepared or what looked so delicious in the store. So you leave it all in the refrigerator and don't eat—and as a result, you feel more tired than ever. As we said above, in order to enhance the effects of the chemotherapy (and to avoid losing so much weight that you're no longer able to tolerate the drugs), you *must* eat. Therefore, you have to break the vicious cycle of fatigue and lack of appetite . The following suggestions won't work for everyone all the time, but they are worth thinking about and trying because they save energy and take advantage of your strengths.

➤ Don't do a huge grocery shopping where you have to carry a dozen bags to the car and then into the house—and then put it all away. Instead, buy a few things at a time (one grocery bag maximum), and when you get home, put away only the perishables. The rest can wait. Or better yet, don't shop at all. Have a family member do it, pay a neighbor's teenager to go to the store for you, and find out which stores in your area deliver. In some major cities, you can even order your groceries online.

➤ Keep all your large and heavy cooking equipment on the countertop so you don't have to crawl into the back of the cupboard every time you want to use the electric mixer or food processor. Your kitchen may look cluttered for a while, but it will be a lot easier on you—and hey, whose kitchen is it, anyway?

➤ Stay off your feet as much as possible. Sit at the kitchen table to prepare food or at the counter on a high stool with a back.

➤ Eat when you have the most energy. For most people, this is the morning. For two reasons, eat as big a breakfast as you can manage. First, it will give you energy for the rest of the day, and second, if your energy dwindles as the day progresses, you might not feel like eating another full meal.

➤ Cook when you have the most energy. Again, this will probably be during the morning. Put on a pot of soup or stew when you feel able to cut up the vegetables, and then all you'll have to do is give it a stir every once in a while until it's done.

➤ If you work during the day and you're the main cook at home, get takeout food for dinner whenever you don't feel up to cooking.

➤ Heat frozen dinners in the microwave when you feel overcome by fatigue. If you find them depressing, take them out of the little plastic dish and put the meal on your best china.

➤ Keep meal planning simple, and take advantage of some of the preparation work the store will do for you. For example, buy salad greens in a bag so you don't have to wash, dry, and tear up lettuce. Buy stew meat in cut-up chunks and chicken parts that are already separated. Buy shrimp and crabmeat already shelled, and get big bags of frozen vegetables that require absolutely no preparation.

Chapter Eleven

Nontraditional Cancer Therapy

Some Alternatives to Traditional Treatment
May Work, but Most Do Not

*L*et's begin with a note about definitions. *Alternative medicine* is by nature unproven. Its practitioners promote its various treatment modalities, such as herbal remedies, anti-neoplastons, and high-dose vitamin therapy, to cure cancer. It is almost always expensive, it is usually not covered by health insurance, and it has no basis in scientific or medical reality.

Complementary medicine, akin to but not the same as alternative medicine, is not promoted to cure cancer. Instead, it is touted as a way to enhance well being, relieve stress, and improve quality of life. Popular treatment modalities include mental imagery, exercise, yoga, and other types of supportive care.

Most forms of alternative healing or alternative medicine are lumped together in an approach called *holistic healing*. The goal of the practitioner is to treat the patient as a whole person rather than as an ailing body part. Theoretically, this is desirable, but with few exceptions, *it is not the way most alternative practitioners practice*. Most make a diagnosis, prescribe a treatment, and demand payment right then and there—a lot like mainstream doctors.

In the September 17, 1998, issue of the *New England Journal of Medicine*, M. Angell and J. Kassirer wrote an editorial called "Alternative Medicine—the Risks of Untested and Unregulated Remedies." They state:

> *What sets most alternative medicine apart is that it has not been scientifically tested and its advocates largely deny the need for such*

testing. By testing, we mean the marshaling of rigorous evidence of safety and efficacy as required by the Food and Drug Administration for the approval of drugs and by the best peer-reviewed medical journals for the publication of research reports. . . . Alternative medicine also distinguishes itself by an ideology that largely ignores biologic mechanisms, often disparaging modern science, and relies on what are purported to be ancient practices and natural remedies (which are seen as somehow being simultaneously more potent and less toxic than conventional medicine). Accordingly, herbs or mixtures of herbs are considered superior to the active compounds isolated in the laboratory.

One philosophy of holistic care is that people are generally healthy (in body and mind) and that we exist in a state of being that seeks balance (*homeostasis*) but is in a constant state of flux. Again, this sounds fine, but if we were so healthy, we wouldn't need to spend money on doctors—holistic, alternative, *or* traditional. And if you have cancer, you're not healthy at all, so the benefits of this theory go right out the window—at least while you have the disease.

Holistic care emphasizes self-healing; that is, the human body exists in a constant state of breakdown and repair. This is true, but it happens without outside intervention. And right now, for you, it is not true at all. Your cancer places you in a state of serious "breakdown." The *only* way you will experience this "repair" is to get treated by a mainstream, highly experienced oncologist. There are times when alternative healing techniques can boost the body's and mind's own powers, but this is rare—and they *cannot* cure cancer.

Many nontraditional healers use the word *energy* when they talk about what they do. They don't mean electric power or rays of sunlight. They seem to refer to some source that human beings have within themselves that can be used for strength, for healing, for power. Whatever this energy is, we all have it, although we call it by different names: soul, will, spirit, essence, anima, breath of life. In any case, you will find it inside yourself, *not* in an alternative healer's office. It cannot be purchased or prescribed.

There also is an approach to alternative healing called *vitalism*, a concept that holds that bodily functions are controlled by a vital principle or life force separate from the forces that explain the laws of physics and chemistry, and that are detectable by scientific instruments. Practitioners of vitalism believe that diseases should be treated by the body's ability to heal itself rather than by treating symptoms.

Again, this sounds lovely, but cancer patients should ask themselves why, if the body has the power to heal itself, a cancer began to grow and metastasize.

Recent Trends

A recent article in the *New England Journal of Medicine* reported that more than a third of the general population surveyed said they use "unconventional therapy," which is defined as medical treatments that are not taught in U.S. medical schools and that are not generally practiced by American physicians. In addition, Americans made 425 million visits to alternative medical practitioners and only 388 million visits to primary care physicians in one recent year. The total cost of alternative therapy was $13.7 billion, 75 percent of which was not reimbursed by health insurance.

These numbers tell a significant story. Americans are willing to spend time and money on healing techniques that are unscientific, unproven, and that make most physicians throw up their hands in horror. Why?

The reasons are numerous and complex. Mainstream (traditional) medicine is expensive and relies on drugs, surgery, and high technology. However, alternative care may be no cheaper if you have to pay for it entirely out of your own pocket, and many such practitioners use or prescribe a variety of pills (most of which have *not* been approved by the Food and Drug Administration), potions, herbs, and mechanical devices. But these treatments differ from what we're used to, which may be one of the appeals.

People complain that traditional medicine is fragmented and that we are shunted from specialist to specialist, which leaves us feeling as if we are traveling on an assembly line. However, in modern medicine, it is impossible to know everything about what ails the human body, and often a specialist is needed. Again, this is the case when you have cancer. While unconventional practitioners tout the advantage of "holistic" healing, an herbalist or a naturopath will not be able to do one thing to treat cancer. At best, you may come out of the office with a recommendation for a healthier diet and some potions to calm your nerves—which may or may not be effective.

People with cancer become frustrated by the length and complexity of the treatment—and sometimes with the inability of mainstream medicine to cure them. This is not rational, but it is understandable. So they rush to alternative healers or the purveyors of quack medicine in the vain hope of a cure. It has been estimated that about 50 percent of all cancer patients use alternative or complementary medicine at some time during—or sometimes in lieu of—mainstream treatment.

Should You Seek Unconventional Treatment?

We cannot recommend specific treatment of any kind, but even if we could, the question is difficult to answer in a general way because so much of alternative therapy is highly individualized. (This is one of the reasons it's so difficult to test.) There are so few scientific studies that it is almost impossible to know if the treatments do any good—or if they do serious harm.

In a 1998 *Journal of the American Medical Association* editorial called "Alternative Medicine Meets Science," P. B. Fontanarosa and G. D. Lundberg made the following comments:

> *There is no alternative medicine. There is only scientifically proven, evidence-based medicine supported by solid data or unproven medicine, for which scientific evidence is lacking. Whether a therapeutic practice is "Eastern" or "Western," is unconventional or mainstream, or involves mind-body techniques or molecular genetics is largely irrelevant except for historical purposes and cultural interest.*

In other words, Fontanarosa and Lundberg argue that either a treatment has been proven to work or it hasn't. It's as simple as that.

Unconventional treatment is probably not for most people, but if you believe strongly in the power of unconventional healing, if you are convinced that you will be helped, and if you are *equally convinced that you will not be harmed*, then you might want to give it a try.

Some Guidelines

If you decide to try an unconventional treatment, do follow these guidelines:

➤ Make sure the treatment enhances your sense of well-being.
➤ Make sure the treatment is based on spiritual, nutritional, and psychological components.

➤ *DO NOT* deny yourself the benefits of proven cancer treatment.

In this way, you may be able to enhance the quality of your life during the time you have cancer.

Some Warnings

Not all unconventional medicine is equally bad—or equally acceptable. Whatever healing techniques or medical interventions you choose, they will be more effective if you cooperate with and encourage the process through your willingness to be healed or cured. Stories abound about people's courage and ability to prevail in the face of "certain" death from cancer.

Some practitioners are well-intentioned and will not hurt you. But there are practitioners all over the place peddling cancer cures that you should stay far, far away from for two major reasons. First, *these cures have no positive medical effect and will do nothing but shrink your wallet*. Second, wasting time and energy on an alternative or natural cure for cancer will prevent you from seeking traditional medical care, which has an excellent chance of helping you.

Unconventional or alternative treatment has become "politically correct" in the past decade or so, but it is not for everyone. Although we strongly urge you to be very wary of patronizing alternative healers for treatment of cancer, if you want to consult one, the following suggestions might protect you from the worst abuses:

➤ Look askance at personal endorsements: "Jane's tumor shrank by 50 percent in three months with such-and-such cancer remedy," or "Dick has been pain free for a year after using the so-and-so machine." Jane and Dick might indeed have a smaller tumor or may feel better, but it's probably not the result of the advertised claim. Personal anecdotes can *never* take the place of scientific testing.

➤ If you feel that an alternative practitioner is trying to hoodwink you or is making ridiculous claims, you're probably right. *Leave the office.*

➤ Don't be fooled by fancy titles or degrees on the wall. Someone either is a physician or is not. Look at the diplomas and license (most states require them to be displayed, and all reputable physicians do it anyway), and if you don't recognize the educational institution or licensing body, ask what the framed certificates mean. If you don't get a straight answer, leave the office.

➤ Make certain you understand all the risks and side effects of the treatment to which you are about to submit. All medical treatment, regardless of who provides it, carries risk, and you have a right to know what it is. If the practitioner tells you that it is "absolutely safe" or "guaranteed to heal," *leave the office. It's a lie.*

➤ If you have to pay for the treatment up front or are required to make a deposit before your appointment, find someone else. Does a restaurant require you to pay for the meal before you eat it?

➤ If a practitioner says that your cancer was caused by faulty nutrition, or can be cured by nutritional supplements, don't believe it. It is simply not true—and it doesn't even make sense.

➤ Beware of pseudomedical jargon and highly nonspecific treatments, such as "detoxification," "chemical balancing," bringing your body "into harmony with nature," or "weakness" of various organs. Ask what these things mean in terms of cancer, and you won't get a sensible answer.

➤ Legitimate medical science is done in collaboration with other scientists, and data are published in reputable medical journals available to you in libraries. In other words, it is an open, public endeavor. "Secret cures" are nothing but quackery.

The Patient's Belief and Participation

All cancer patients must participate in their own treatment in order to get the best results. That is, you have to show up for the chemotherapy appointments, no matter how much you don't want to; you need to submit to the follow-up tests and evaluations, no matter how unpleasant and time-consuming; and you have to put up with the side effects and do whatever is suggested to minimize them, no matter how horrid they make you feel. Perhaps most important, you have to force yourself to have a positive attitude, to believe that the treatment will work and that you will get better.

In alternative medicine, the patient plays an even greater role, primarily because belief in the treatment's efficacy has to substitute for scientific proof. Many alternative practitioners talk about the patient's belief system, which may or may not have a basis in an established religion. They talk about spirituality, in all its individualistic connotations, and the positive "energy" that arises from spirituality and belief in the treatment that is being undertaken. They also talk about the relationship between the patient and the caregiver—the patient's belief in the healing power and sympathy of the health care provider.

If all this sounds warm and fuzzy and nice, but lacking the meat of scientific and medical efficacy, you're right. There is no harm in having positive thoughts about a treatment (or the person providing it), and spiritual faith certainly never harmed anyone unless it turned into religious zealotry. *But it isn't enough.* The treatment has to have worked on others, or it has to have shown enough real promise that the practitioner is willing to submit it to the exacting standards of provable clinical safety and efficacy.

Mainstream Versus Alternative Cancer Therapy
Dialogue at a Conference
In late summer 1998, a conference was held to see if mainstream and alternative practitioners could work together to provide comprehensive, integrated cancer treatment. (At the conference, which was held in Washington, D.C., the word *complementary* was used as well as *alternative*.) The conference was cosponsored by the Center for Mind-Body Medicine in Washington, D.C.; the Office of Alternative Medicine at the National Institutes of Health; and the Medical School and School of Nursing of the University of Texas Health Science Center at Houston. A year later, a second such conference took place.

According to James S. Gordon, M.D., clinical professor of psychiatry and family medicine at Georgetown University in Washington and Director of the Center for Mind-Body Medicine, the conference was not about alternative versus traditional medicine. He explained, "It's about what's most useful for people. Let's open up the lens; let's all learn from each other and look at the evidence for efficacy together."

Robert E. Wittes, M.D., director of the Division of Cancer Treatment and Diagnosis at the National Cancer Institute (NCI), said, "The integration of everything we know is a noble goal. It's philosophically impossible to disagree with it in principle, but for the goal of integrative treatment to be achieved, practitioners from mainstream and complementary medicine must have respect for the scientific evidence that supports claims of efficacy. The evidence is everything."

On a more conciliatory note, he added, "We need to stop fighting about where our hypotheses come from and start arguing about evidence. Only then will we make progress." He noted that this belief is becoming more widely shared in the cancer community. "The traditionalists are now less likely to dismiss complementary and alternative medicine out of hand. They seem to care more about whether a treatment works, rather than the credentials of the person providing it. We are learning how to separate the wheat from the chaff with people who are knowledgeable about both mainstream and complementary medicine."

Shortly before the second meeting, and after the demise of the National Institutes of Health Office of Alternative Medicine, NCI established, as part of the director's office, the National Center for Complementary and Alternative Medicine. It exists, primarily as a result of political pressure, to determine if there is scientific validity to claims of alternative treatments for cancer. So far, no such proof has been established, although there are a few clinical trials in the planning stages. Dr. Wittes lauded the new center, but he noted a number of barriers to integrative cancer treatment:

➤ Some of the hypotheses of alternative therapies are incompatible with the bedrock principles of Western science that are ingrained in mainstream physicians.

➤ Many alternative treatments are complex programs with multiple interwoven components. There is nothing wrong with this in and of itself, but mainstream scientists are used to dissecting components of therapy and testing them for safety and efficacy in clinical trials. The complexity of an alternative approach makes this difficult or impossible. A great many alternative therapies rely on "extreme individualization" of therapy so that treatment becomes patient-specific. With such an emphasis, it is difficult to test the therapy.

It was the consensus of the mainstream physicians and scientists at the meeting that all cancer therapy must stand the test of peer-reviewed scientific evaluation. That is, other scientists must be able to scrutinize the data and replicate it in their own laboratories and with their own patients. David S. Rosenthal, M.D., president of the American Cancer Society and professor of medicine at Harvard Medical School, urged cancer patients to remain in the care of mainstream physicians who use standard, evidence-based therapies. He also urged cancer patients to tell their physicians if they are using alternative treatments.

Further Dialogue at a Research Meeting

In the spring of 1999, more than 20,000 people attended a meeting of the American Society for Clinical Oncology (ASCO), the most important and prestigious cancer research organization in the country. At the meeting, which was cosponsored by ASCO and the American Cancer Society, a symposium was given on complementary and alternative medicine (CAM) in cancer care.

Although, as one might expect, the scientists who participated in and attended the symposium expressed a skeptical view of CAM, there was a general feeling that CAM should not be dismissed out of hand. This was best summed up by Arnold Relman, M.D., editor-in-chief emeritus of the *New England Journal of Medicine* and professor emeritus of medicine and social medicine at Harvard Medical School. He said, "CAM is not based on modern scientific views of nature, and is not validated by objective evidence or the gold standard of the randomized clinical trial."

He argued that physicians should tell their patients the truth: that most CAM is unproven and unlikely to be beneficial. However, he added, "Patients do need support and should not be deprived of hope. Physicians should not recommend, endorse, or approve an unproven medicine, but CAM could be considered when all medical therapeutic modalities have been exhausted, and a fully informed patient wants CAM and it will not interfere with medical therapy." Dr. Relman added that the medical community should keep an open mind as evidence becomes available, but the burden of proof rests with the proponent of an alternative therapy.

Impending Clinical Trials

As in all areas of medical research, funds are limited for complementary and alternative medicine clinical trials. Therefore, the NCI administration needs to be careful about how to best allocate resources. Dr. Wittes said, "We need to see evidence of a claim's credibility before we fund a clinical trial, and we would like to find some scientific and medical opportunity—that is, if it can be tied to existing scientific knowledge, for instance the possible anti-cancer properties of green tea. We also feel there should be a certain amount of public interest in the treatment modality."

He listed a few planned NCI-sponsored clinical trials, or ideas for trials, most of which will take place at the M. D. Anderson Cancer Center in Houston, which has been designated as a research site by the Office of Complementary and Alternative Medicine:

➤ A Phase III trial of shark cartilage (sharks never get cancer) plus chemotherapy in lung and prostate cancers will get underway shortly.

➤ Green tea, polyphenols, selenium, and Newcastle disease virus may act as cancer preventives, and it may be possible to test this hypothesis in clinical trials.

➤ Melatonin, which has immunologic, anti-oxidant, anti-tumor, and anti-estogenic effects, with a combination chemotherapy regimen (CHOP), is being tested in a Phase III trial in patients with lymphoma. It is thought that melatonin can reduce thrombocytopenia and other side effects of chemotherapy.

➤ A study of mistletoe, in combination with fluorouracil and leucovorin, is being considered for treatment of colorectal cancer. Mistletoe has long been used in Germany to reduce pain, stimulate the immune system, and improve quality of life.

➤ Oleander may stabilize some types of cancer and is being studied.

Nutrition and Cancer

Many alternative practitioners use nutrients in their concoctions to treat cancer. They consist mainly of high doses of vitamins and minerals and herbs. Not one of these treatments has been proved to cure cancer, but mainstream medical research has found some evidence regarding the following:

> A high-fat diet tends to promote breast, colon, and prostate cancers. Note that this does not prove a direct cause-and-effect relationship.
> Dietary fiber *may* prevent colorectal cancer.
> Cruciferous vegetables (cabbage, broccoli, cauliflower, and Brussels sprouts) have anti-cancer properties.
> Ellagic acid, found in raspberries, *may* help prevent colon cancer, especially in people with a hyperactive colon.
> Selenium *may* prevent prostate cancer.

Complementary Therapy

None of the following treatments can cure cancer or should even be attempted as a treatment for the disease. But cancer creates a number of symptoms related to, but not part of, the disease, such as pain. Complementary techniques may help alleviate some of these symptoms.

Acupuncture

Acupuncture is one of the most widely accepted alternative therapies, and some mainstream physicians even recommend it for patients in pain. In 1997, an FDA advisory committee acknowledged that acupuncture does indeed have therapeutic value. This may not sound like a big deal, but it is. The FDA is an extremely cautious agency; you can feel confident that a treatment modality that receives its imprimatur is safe and effective. Moreover, you are now more likely to get your health insurance carrier to reimburse you for acupuncture.

Acupuncture, which originated in China more than 2,000 years ago, involves the insertion of very fine needles into certain points on the skin, the purpose of which is to unblock or balance the flow of life force throughout the body. Some traditional physicians, while acknowledging the efficacy of acupuncture, attribute its effects to the release of endorphin, a naturally occurring chemical that acts as a pain reliever.

The only real way in which acupuncture can have a positive effect on cancer is pain relief. If you are in severe pain and do not want to take as many analgesic drugs as you have been prescribed, you might consider an acupuncturist.

Chiropractic Spinal Manipulation

Chiropractic spinal manipulation has been pooh-poohed by traditional medicine for decades, but it may be a good treatment for some types of back pain. However, it is NOT a good treatment if you have bone cancer or metastasis to the bone. In those cases, *spinal manipulation may cause bone fracture.*

The theory behind chiropractic treatment is that back problems (and other body dysfunction) stem from a misalignment of the vertebrae and that physical adjustment can get them back in place. If this is indeed your problem, you may find relief in a chiropractor's office, but you will NOT find relief for anything else. The spinal column has *no causative connection* with any other ailment, including cancer.

If you think your backaches are caused by stress, chiropractic treatment may help. It can't hurt, and you will soon find out if it helps you. One further word of warning: do *not* seek this type of treatment if you have a herniated disk. Manipulating the vertebrae in the presence of this condition can do serious damage to the spinal nerves. Some health insurance carriers cover chiropractic treatment, so check with your agent.

Massage

Massage is a way to create deep relaxation. In addition, it can improve joint range of motion, improve blood circulation, and generally enhance a sense of well being. Be warned, though, that if you have blood clots, phlebitis, a skin disease, contusions, or infections, you should NOT get a massage, which can exacerbate them.

Naturopathy

Naturopathy emphasizes a healthy lifestyle (good nutrition, no smoking, stress reduction, and the like), but its belief that many illnesses can be cured by purging the body of impurities is bunk. A naturopath can do absolutely *nothing* to treat cancer, and you are better off buying a book on nutrition than shelling out your hard-earned money (which will not be reimbursed by your health insurer) for naturopathy.

Herbal Medicine

The use of herbs as medicines is a very "iffy" business. Herbal medicine uses various plant leaves, stems, roots, and seeds to cure ills, and its practice is as old as human life on earth. Because herbal remedies contain such complex ingredients, there is no way to accurately test them for safety and efficacy, but some have been known to make people feel better—or think they feel better, which is much the same thing. Moreover, some well-tested and commonly accepted medications started out as herbal remedies, such as digitalis for heart disease, rauwolfia for hypertension—and aspirin.

Some alternative practitioners claim that cancer is caused by "impure blood" and suggest a variety of purifying herbs ranging from alfalfa to yellowdock. *None* of these cures cancer.

The FDA does not regulate herbal medicine, and there is no way to know what they really contain. Therefore, a good rule of thumb is: *If you can buy it in a health food store, beware of it.* Nevertheless, some cancer patients find that herbal and other remedies can ease symptoms. For example, vitamin E provides relief of the frequency and severity of the hot flashes that often accompany hormonal treatment for breast cancer. Although it is hard to get enough vitamin E from natural sources to create a therapeutic effect, foods that are good sources of the vitamin are wheat germ, wheat germ oil, safflower oil, whole grain breads and cereals, peanuts, walnuts, filberts, and almonds. A more efficient way to get a therapeutic dose of vitamin E is to take it in pill form: 800 to 1,600 units a day.

Garlic and other herbs, such as chamomile, catnip, hops, and passion flower, can be soothing and relaxing and are said to reduce stress. Taken in moderation (an occasional cup of tea), they probably can't hurt you, and they may even help.

If you do take herbal remedies, read the label carefully and try to find out if the manufacturer is reputable. The FDA Web site *(www.fda.gov)* will provide a link to the Division of Over-the-Counter Drugs, where you can get more information. Also, don't be surprised if the directions tell you to take six or eight or even ten pills at a time. Herbs are far less purified than the chemicals we know as medications, and the pills often contain a proportionately larger amount of binder such as cellulose, starch, sugar, and other pharmacologically inactive ingredients.

Treatments that Can Cause Serious Harm
Chelation Therapy

Chelation therapy, an intravenous infusion of chemicals designed to flush metal out of the body, is *highly dangerous*. While practitioners of this therapy claim that it is an acceptable alternative to cardiac bypass surgery—some even tout it as a cancer treatment—the *only* legitimate use for chelation therapy is to treat lead poisoning. Even then, it should be done only in a hospital (usually in the emergency room) under the care of traditional physicians experienced in its use. If you find yourself in the office of someone who recommends chelation therapy as a treatment or cure for cancer, make tracks for the door in a hurry.

Dietary Supplements

Many people believe in taking dietary supplements in addition to (rarely instead of) traditional cancer chemotherapy. However, certain kinds of dietary supplements, if taken in sufficient quantity, can kill. At best, they do nothing or cause illness. For example, taking amino acids will not build muscle, increase intelligence, or treat insomnia. Large doses of vitamin A will not improve your vision; rather they can cause liver damage and birth defects. Megadoses of vitamin B6 have been associated with nerve damage, and too much niacin causes nausea, vomiting, diarrhea, and liver damage. And the once-popular L-tryptophan, touted to relieve insomnia, killed 387 people, and hundreds of others suffered from crippling muscle pain.

The FDA does not guarantee the safety and efficacy of any of these dietary supplements and is trying to crack down on their manufacture. It is against the law to sell any product for which a health claim is made unless it has been approved by the FDA, but manufacturers have devised a number of ways to evade FDA inspectors and federal marshals.

For some reason, some cancer patients believe that dietary supplements in the form of vitamins and minerals can increase the effects of chemotherapy. This is not true, and even if you suffer no physical harm, you will have wasted your money. If you eat a well-balanced diet, you will get all the vitamins and minerals you need.

Instrumentation

Alternative health practitioners sometimes try to snow people with a variety of electrical and mechanical devices that claim to have magical healing powers. They prey especially on cancer patients, who are usually more scared and vulnerable than other patients. Federal marshals seize these products when and where they can, but as always, there are more bad guys than good guys in the criminal arena, so there are still thousands of these machines out there in "doctors'" offices.

High Colonics

High colonic irrigation, a procedure in which as many as 20 gallons of water are pumped into the intestines through a tube inserted into the rectum, has been prescribed by alternative practitioners to cleanse the body of its impurities. But the body's own organs—liver, kidneys, and intestines—are designed to do this job, so leave them alone and let them get on with it! For people with cancer, a colonic irrigation could be especially dangerous because it can interfere with the rate of excretion of drugs, as well as with the rate of absorption of nutrients.

Other "Treatments"

In addition to "purification of the blood" with various herbal remedies, alternative practitioners recommend extremely weird treatments for cancer. Some are harmful; others are just useless. Here are a few examples. *Stay away from all of them.*

- ➤ Eschewing all meat, many other proteins, and synthetic foods and eating only organic foods
- ➤ Speeding up peristalsis by eating laxative foods (prunes, figs, raisins, and the like) and using laxative herbs
- ➤ Chlorophyll to slow the growth of cancerous tumors
- ➤ Chlorophyll and/or coffee retention enemas (holding the solution in the rectum for a half hour or more) to "detoxify" the system
- ➤ Moving to a warm, unpolluted climate
- ➤ Soaking in a tub of warm salted water to draw out toxins
- ➤ Hair analysis to determine the presence of toxic heavy metals
- ➤ Poly-ZYM-023 enzymes to break down the "protective shield" around a tumor
- ➤ Megadoses of vitamin A to minimize liver involvement
- ➤ Raw thymus gland to increase lymphocytes

Treatments that Are Useless but Harmless

> ➤ *Aromatherapy* is an ancient Chinese form of herbal medicine that claims to cure various ills with aromatic plant oils, which may smell pleasant and put one in a better mood. However, aromatherapy does nothing for health.

> ➤ *Bee pollen* has been promoted for treatment of obesity, high blood pressure, arthritis, and—more recently and with lots of publicity—multiple sclerosis. There is no evidence to support any health claims for bee pollen.

> ➤ *Crystals* may look pretty on a chain around your neck or dangling from your earlobes, but they exert no aura and have no effect on the body.

> ➤ *Reflexology* is massage that claims to treat illness and keep the life force in balance—whatever that means. *Foot massage* has been touted to govern energy channels—whatever they are. A nice massage is relaxing and a good stress reducer, but it has no other health benefits.

> ➤ *Homeopathy* is a technique that treats disease with tiny doses of natural substances that in larger amounts would cause the same symptoms. The theory is that illness is caused by a disturbance in the body's "vital force," and that these substances help the body heal itself by boosting natural defenses. There is no evidence that homeopathy does any good, but the substances are given in such a small amount that they probably won't hurt. There is no logical reason to believe that homeopathy would have any effect at all on cancer because the disease is not caused by an external substance.

Unproven Treatments

Unproven is a diplomatic way to talk about treatments that fall somewhere between absolute bunk and possibly helpful. The American Cancer Society (ACS) defines unproven treatments as "those diagnostic tests or therapeutic modalities which are promoted for general use in cancer prevention, diagnosis, or treatment and which are, on the basis of careful review by scientists and/or clinicians, not deemed proven nor recommended for current use."

These treatments are also called *unorthodox* or *questionable*, and because they have not been subjected to scientific scrutiny (or have failed such scrutiny), the ACS does not endorse their use. Although the society does not come right out and say, "Steer clear of these treatments," you should be very, very leery of them.

Nutritional and *metabolic therapies* are promoted on the theory that cancer is the result of the buildup of toxic and waste materials in the body that interfere with metabolism and healing. The following treatments comprise efforts to detoxify the body and eliminate wastes. Most of them rely on nutritional factors, megadoses of vitamins and minerals, large-volume enemas (coyly called "internal cleansing"), and a spiritual and emotional component.

> ➤ *The Gerson diet*, or *treatment*, was developed by Max Gerson, M.D., to treat his own migraine headaches. He expanded it to treat arthritis and then cancer, and by the time he emigrated from Germany to the United States in 1938 and passed his medical boards in New York in 1939, Gerson concentrated only on treating cancer, which he believed is a degenerative disease caused by the failure of the immune system to produce an "allergic inflammation," or healing reaction. Gerson's diet concentrated on low-sodium, high-potassium foods; huge amounts of fresh fruit and vegetable juices; iron supplements; liver extract injections; pancreatic enzymes; other supplements; and coffee enemas to rid the body of toxins and to improve general health. Several people have become seriously ill or have died as a result of the Gerson regimen, so stay away from it.

> ➤ *Kelly metabolic therapy*, also known as *Kelly ecology therapy*, was developed by William Donald Kelly, an orthodontist who had pancreatic cancer. He believed that cancer was caused by a deficiency of a pancreatic enzyme and diminished protein metabolism. The diet includes 25 nutritional supplements and pancreatic enzymes (some patients have to take up to 300 pills a day), detoxifying treatments such as coffee enemas, exercise, fasting and purging, chiropractic and osteopathic treatments, and a spiritual component to "purify the emotions." The diet is vegetarian, and patients are instructed to avoid white flour, tea, coffee, chocolate, liquor, and white rice. In 1970, Kelly was ordered not to practice medicine (remember, he was an orthodontist), and most medical reviewers found his regimen

useless. Today, the regimen touted by Nicholas Gonzalez, M.D., is similar to Kelly metabolic therapy—without the neurological and spiritual components.

➤ *Manner metabolic cancer therapy* was designed by Harold W. Manner, Ph.D., a biologist who thought that cancer was the result of a weak immune system. His regimen consists of a pretreatment hair and blood test to measure mineral imbalances, a special diet, combinations of laetrile and megadoses of vitamins and minerals, and the much beloved coffee enemas. Laetrile is a dangerous substance that can cause death from cyanide poisoning, and there is a wide variety of side effects from megadoses of vitamins and minerals, some of them life-threatening.

➤ The *macrobiotic diet* was developed in Japan by George Ohsawa and consists mostly of organically grown vegetables, unprocessed cereals and grains, seafood, and soy-based miso and tamari broth. It is an extremely popular alternative cancer treatment and is an important component of the Zen Buddhist way of life. To live on a pure macrobiotic diet is extremely complex, and directions for food preparation are highly specific. The regimen can lead to serious nutritional deficiencies, which is dangerous for anyone but especially so for cancer patients.

➤ *Hoxsey herbal treatment*, devised by Harry Hoxsey, is a tonic that is purported to contain potassium iodide, licorice, red clover, buckthorn bark, pokeweed root, and other herbs and minerals. The tonic is believed to cause the elimination of toxins that poison the body. In 1960, the FDA banned shipping the Hoxsey tonic across state lines, so to all intents and purposes, it is illegal in the United States.

Other useless potions and remedies abound. Some are popular for a while and then fall into disuse or disrepute even among those on the fringes of alternative cancer therapy. Here are a few of the most popular ones out of the many in current use:

➤ Laetrile has been around for years. It is derived from amygdalin found in apricot pits and was first used as cancer treatment by Ernst Krebs, Sr., M.D., in the 1950s. Krebs and his followers claimed that laetrile destroys cancer cells and relieves pain. It does not. Not only does it not cure cancer, it breaks down in the body to form cyanide, which can cause a number of serious side effects, including death.

➤ Vitamin C (ascorbic acid) has been highly touted by Ewan Cameron, a Scottish surgeon, and Linus Pauling, an American Nobel laureate in chemistry, as an effective treatment for cancer. They believed that it would slow progression of the disease by inhibiting tumor growth and by strengthening tissue adjacent to the tumor to make it more resistant to metastasis. Randomized double-blind studies funded by the NCI found that vitamin C contained no therapeutic value when compared to a placebo. What's more, it caused serious side effects such as vomiting and diarrhea. Moreover, excess amounts of vitamin C may even promote tumor growth.

➤ *Immuno-augmentive therapy* (IAT), developed by biologist Lawrence Burton, Ph.D., is designed to beef up the immune system because Burton believes that cancer is caused by a breakdown of that system. Although there are elements of rationality in this theory, there is no reason to believe that IAT—which consists of the patient's own "tumor antibodies" and "tumor complement," as well as "deblocking protein" from healthy people—is an effective treatment for cancer.

➤ *Antineoplaston therapy* is one of the most controversial alternative therapies, primarily because its developer, Stanislaw Burzynski, M.D., Ph.D., has been able to convince some scientists and several politicians that his treatment has merit. Burzynski believes that substances called antineoplastons (composed of peptides and amino acid derivatives), which are part of a biomedical defense system, correct defective cells and restore them to normal. Burzynski provides his treatment at a private clinic, and in 1991, he was able to convince the NCI to review a series of his claimed successes. The NCI found that in seven cases of advanced brain cancer, antineoplaston therapy *may* have had some anti-tumor activity.

➤ *Oxygen therapy* (also known as *hyperoxygenation, oxymedicine,* or *bio-oxidative therapy*) is based on the belief that cancer is caused by an oxygen deficiency. The theory was developed by German Nobel Laureate Otto Warburg, M.D., who said that the way to treat cancer is to expose malignant cells to high levels of oxygen. The treatment is given by administering ozone or hydrogen peroxide by a variety of routes, including ozone enemas. There is no reason to believe that oxygen therapy has *any* positive effect on cancer, and it may even damage healthy tissue.

➤ *Dimethyl sulfoxide* (DMSO) is an industrial solvent used to treat a variety of diseases, cancer among them. However, it is approved by the FDA *only* for treatment of interstitial cystitis, a bladder condition. It is often used in conjunction with metabolic therapy, laetrile, and other alternative treatments. Regardless of how it is used, alone or in combination, DMSO has *no* effect on cancer.

➤ The *Revici method* of "biologically guided" chemotherapy was developed by Emanuel Revici, M.D., who ran a private hospital in New York, where he was chief of oncology. The hospital was convicted of Medicaid fraud, and Revici himself had his medical license temporarily suspended. Biologically guided chemotherapy is purported to correct imbalances in bodily agents such as lipid alcohols, zinc, lithium, fatty acids, selenium, and others. Several reputable medical institutions have attempted to objectively test the Revici method, but Revici would not agree to any of the proposed evaluation methods, and no one has ever been able to find any evidence of tumor regression as a result of the treatment.

➤ *Livingston-Wheeler therapy*, according to its developer, Virginia Livingston-Wheeler, M.D., is a combination of a vaccine made from each patient's own bacteria (extracted from blood and excreta), other established vaccines, gamma globulin, sheep spleen extract, liver extracts, and other components. In addition, patients are subjected to hot water, lemon juice, or coffee enemas and doses of castor oil and Epsom salts. Megadoses of vitamins and minerals also are given. Livingston-Wheeler insists on a strict vegetarian diet that is eaten mostly raw. Again, there is no evidence of efficacy in Livingston-Wheeler therapy.

Chapter Twelve

Paying for Chemotherapy

It's Expensive, but That's Why You Have Insurance

Health Insurance

Cancer can be an expensive disease, so if you don't have health insurance, you will have serious problems.

If you work, you will probably buy it as part of your employer's benefit package. If your employer does not provide it, if you are self-employed, or if you are ineligible to be a dependent of your spouse's policy (or are unmarried), buy a policy yourself.

If you are one of the more than 44 million Americans who does not now have health insurance, and if you can afford it, you have two choices about *how* you buy it: you can go it alone and buy an individual policy, or you can join an organization and become eligible for its group health benefits. The only problem is that if you don't have health insurance now and you are diagnosed with cancer, any policy you purchase will most likely carry pre-existing condition restrictions. You have two essential choices here: don't mention the cancer when you apply for coverage—and be prepared to pay the very stiff penalties if the carrier finds out that you lied; or be honest at the outset and prepare to put up a fight (and likely lose because the rules are clearly stated in the policy) when the carrier refuses to pay all claims for cancer treatment. The bottom line is that if you don't have health insurance when you are diagnosed with cancer, you're pretty much out of luck about having someone else pick up the tab for the treatment.

Types of Health Insurance
Fee for Service
With *fee-for-service* insurance, sometimes called *traditional* or *conventional plan* health insurance, you pay a premium and then some portion of your health care expenses is reimbursed. The size of the portion and the type of expenses reimbursed vary widely depending on the plan purchased and the amount of the deductible. In a fee-for-service plan, the health care provider first bills the insurance company and then bills the patient for whatever is not covered (called *balance billing*)—unless the health insurance company specifically prohibits the provider from doing this. With *fee-for-service* insurance, you choose whatever health practitioner you want to see.

Health Maintenance Organizations
Health maintenance organizations (HMOs) are managed care insurance plans that an individual or a family joins as a dues-paying member for a flat monthly or quarterly fee. The member receives almost all health care at little additional cost. Most HMOs charge a per-visit fee in order to discourage unnecessary trips to the doctor. An HMO insists that you use one of its staff physicians as your primary care physician (PCP), who is also known as the gatekeeper. The gatekeeper then refers you to a specialist if he or she thinks you require it.

With this type of plan, your choice of a health care practitioner is severely limited. Health maintenance organizations are extremely concerned about keeping health care costs down, and this is why many are loath to send you to a specialist. However, this situation has been improving in recent years because of all the adverse publicity from patients who would have benefited from specialist care.

If you do choose an HMO, research the company very carefully. Make certain it has been around for a while, that it is financially solvent, and that its physicians have good medical backgrounds and are well thought of in the medical community.

Preferred Provider Organizations
A *preferred provider organization* (PPO) is another type of controlled managed care plan whereby physicians and other health care providers arrange with an insurer to discount their fees. Providers are then paid by the insurer, with patients paying a per-visit fee. If you

are a member of a PPO, you receive full coverage if you choose a physician from the preferred list. If you choose an "outside" physician (not one of the preferred providers), you will pay most of the bill yourself. You also may be penalized by losing future benefits.

Tiered Plans

Tiered plans provide a kind of cafeteria of health insurance services, with various levels of choice: HMO, PPO, or fee-for-service. Each level has a different premium structure, a different amount of patient responsibility, and a different amount of choice regarding health care providers. This is the way to have the most freedom of choice, but it also is the most confusing, and it has many rules and regulations that you have to keep straight.

Medicare and Medicaid

Medicare is a federal health insurance program, enacted by an amendment to the Social Security Act, that provides hospital and medical care coverage for people age 65 and older, as well as for some individuals who have been disabled and who have received Social Security benefits for more than 24 months. Medicare is a government entitlement for which you have been paying taxes. It is *not* charity. Part A covers inpatient hospitalization, some skilled nursing care, part-time home health care, and some hospice care. Part B covers physicians' services, outpatient care, x-rays, and laboratory tests, as well as limited coverage for medical equipment such as wheelchairs and hospital beds.

Medicare Part A, for which you do not pay a premium, is administered by the Health Care Financing Administration (HCFA) through private insurers called intermediaries. Part B is directed by HCFA and is funded by a monthly premium, which is deducted from your monthly Social Security check.

Medigap insurance is sold privately through health insurance carriers and covers the 20 percent of Medicare coinsurance for which you are responsible. The various types of Medigap policies vary widely in coverage, so read the fine print before you sign on the dotted line.

Medicaid is a joint federal-state program, also created by the Social Security Act, that provides health services (inpatient care, outpatient services, diagnostic testing, drugs, skilled nursing facility care, and home health care) for people who live at or below the federal poverty level and have no other way to pay for health care. If you have no health insurance when you are diagnosed with cancer and if you cannot afford to pay for the care yourself, a hospital social worker will help you apply for Medicaid. Eligibility requirements and services provided vary from state to state. It too is funded by tax revenues.

Coverage Issues

Except for the pre-existing condition issue if you purchase health insurance after you have been diagnosed with cancer, there should be no problem about covering the costs of the disease. Each carrier has its own rules—some more stringent than others. However, in this day and age of adversarial relationships between health insurance carriers and their clients, anything can happen, so be aware of the following potential pitfalls:

> ➤ The *effective date* of the policy. Did you just purchase it? Have you or your spouse recently changed jobs and are thus subject to a waiting period for the insurance to kick in? If so, you will not be covered until the effective date.
> ➤ The amount of your *deductible*. If it's high, you may want to consider lowering it. However, the price of your premiums will go up, so this move may or may not be cost-effective.
> ➤ The *stop-loss ceiling*. This is the amount you have to pay out-of-pocket until the insurance begins to pay 100 percent of all covered expenses. A stop loss is not the same as a deductible, and it will be stated in the policy contract.
> ➤ The *amount of expenses* your policy actually covers. Most people are unpleasantly surprised to find out that up to a certain point (the stop loss), insurance covers only a certain percentage of all claims. The usual rate is 80 percent or 90 percent, but it could be as low as 50 percent.
> ➤ The *types of care* covered. All policies pay for acute hospital care and all that entails, as well as much outpatient care, diagnostic tests, and laboratory services. But as a cancer patient, you may need other services, such as a home health aide, and your pharmacy bill may be enormous (check right

now to see if you have *prescription drug coverage*). Find out if home nurses or home health aides are covered, as well as care at skilled nursing or convalescent homes. If they're not, start to budget for that possible expense.

➤ The physicians and other health care *providers* you can use. If you have fee-for-service insurance, this shouldn't be a problem, but if you are a member of an HMO or a PPO, you need to know who is covered and who is not so you can factor this information into your choice of specialists.

➤ The *lifetime maximum* of what an insurer will reimburse. Do you have one? Cancer is an expensive disease, and you may have a recurrence some years down the road—which will be more expensive because as time passes, health care costs increase.

➤ The rules about *denial of claims*. When you are diagnosed with cancer and the big bills start showing up in the insurance company's computer, you will probably be assigned to a case manager, usually a nurse or social worker. This person's job is not only to keep costs down (although insurers generally deny this function) but to act as a liaison among health care providers, patients (you), and the insurer. Be sure you find out from your case manager which claims will definitely be paid and which might be denied. In addition to the presence of a pre-existing condition, there are reasons why an insurer will deny a claim: the benefit isn't covered in the policy; you have chosen a provider not authorized by the policy; the treatment is investigational (this once-blanket denial has been relaxed somewhat); the treatment is off label (it is approved by the FDA but not for your condition); and nonpayment of premiums—in other words, your policy has been canceled by default.

Chemotherapy raises the potential for denial of health insurance coverage. Most likely, as long as you are receiving standard treatment for a particular cancer, you will have no trouble with the claims department. However, if you are receiving an investigational drug, or if your oncologist prescribes an off-label use, you may have a fight on your hands.

Using COBRA When Changing Jobs

The Consolidated Omnibus Budget Reconciliation Act (COBRA) is a federal law that protects you (and thus your health insurance) when you leave your job, whether you quit or were fired, so that for 18 months, or until you find another job with health insurance benefits, you may continue to participate with full coverage in the health insurance plan of the job you left. You will have to pay the premiums yourself and the carrier (health insurance company) may charge you up to 2 percent more than it charges the employer. Even so, this is always cheaper than buying an individual policy.

Once you leave your job, you have 60 days to sign up for COBRA benefits, but it is best to do it right away. Even if you are moving on to another job immediately, take the COBRA benefits; there may be a waiting period of one to six months before you are eligible for health insurance benefits on your new job. Even if you are eligible right away, what if you fall and break your leg over the weekend between the old job and the new one?

If you are disabled (and a diagnosis of cancer almost always constitutes a legal disability even if you are not on crutches or in a wheelchair), your COBRA coverage can be extended to 29 months. If after 18 months, you have not found a job, you may be eligible for something called a *conversion policy*. This means that when your COBRA coverage runs out, the carrier will offer to cover you on the same policy—at a much larger premium, of course. About 35 states require insurers to offer conversion policies. When the offer is made, you have 30 days to respond.

Managed Care

Everyone has heard the term *managed care* by now, but not everyone knows what it means. In addition, almost everyone hates managed care, but most people don't know exactly why they have such strong negative feelings. Managed care is the most rapidly growing segment of the health care payment system in the United States—and one of the most complicated.

HMOs are the purest form of managed care, although all health insurance plans now use some type of managed care system. More than 70 million Americans are enrolled in HMOs, and 95 percent of all employee health care benefits are under some type of managed care. In addition, Medicare and Medicaid are moving toward managed care payment systems.

Although managed care is a complex system of paying for health care, it basically means that someone is interposed between patients and health care providers. This someone has the authority to place restrictions on how and from whom patients may receive services and what services are to be provided in any given situation.

Moreover, this someone is almost never your health professional; it is usually an employee of an insurance company or a health maintenance organization. In very broad strokes, here's how it works: you go to your physician, who makes a decision about the type of health care you require. But that decision is not final; unless it is an emergency, your health insurance company will have to approve what the physician wants to do. However, even if your physician makes the final decision about the type of care you need, the managed care organization is always looking over his or her shoulder to keep track of practice patterns—and how much they cost.

In reality, things aren't as bad as this makes it sound. Physicians don't have to make a phone call for every little thing they do because insurance companies have established lists of what they believe are appropriate procedures and treatments for various ailments. These are the things for which the carrier will reimburse you or your physician or other health care provider. For other, out-of-the-ordinary procedures or treatments, you will need to obtain approval from the carrier. It's a nuisance, and that's what everyone—providers and their patients—hates.

However, managed care was instituted for a reason, and it has had some positive fallout. American consumers of health care benefit because they are not subjected to unnecessary tests and treatments. All procedures carry risk and often have serious side effects. The less we are exposed to unnecessary risk, the better off we are, and the better off we are for not having to pay for something we didn't need in the first place.

Health care costs in the United States have been escalating beyond all reason, far outstripping all rates of inflation. In addition, there are about 44 million Americans who have no health insurance at all (not even Medicare or Medicaid) and who have to pay for everything out of their own pockets—or go without care.

One of the reasons why health care costs so much is that so many physicians prescribe inappropriate and unnecessary procedures and treatments. They do this for two major reasons: plain old greed, and a perceived need to practice *defensive medicine*—to perform every diagnostic test and procedure they can think of in an effort to prove they have done everything reasonable and possible in case of a medical malpractice lawsuit.

The first motivation needs no explanation, but you may not know what defensive medicine is. The incidence of medical malpractice lawsuits has escalated so dramatically in the past few decades that physicians are perpetually terrified of being sued, so they perform diagnostic tests and procedures in an effort to cover all bases, and to prove to the plaintiff's lawyers that they did everything reasonable and possible in the care of the patient suing.

Medical malpractice suits, both reasonable and frivolous, have reached epidemic proportions, and health insurance companies have had to foot the bill for these defensive (and usually medically unnecessary) procedures. While they have no way to control who sues a physician, they do have control over what they will and will not reimburse, so they have been clamping down and instituting much more stringent reimbursement policies.

Today, if physicians do a few office procedures in an attempt to diagnose cancer, order a series of outpatient diagnostic tests, and prescribe standard chemotherapy, the insurance carrier will reimburse with no questions asked. But if a physician wants patients to have a stress test in the absence of cardiac symptoms or a brain scan when they have not complained of anything wrong with their head, the carrier will say, "No way!" Those tests would be unnecessary and inappropriate.

Insurers manage health care costs in four general ways.

> ➤ Physicians and other providers are given financial incentives to use fewer services and to discourage patients from overusing services. For cancer patients, this could mean that your primary oncologist might discourage you from seeing another specialist once the diagnosis is made and treatment has begun.
> ➤ Managed care organizations designate certain providers who will give necessary care at the least cost; the practice patterns

of these providers are closely monitored by the organization, especially the number of referrals to specialists.

➤ Insurance policies control and limit the services for which a managed care organization will pay. This means that if you want to go to a pain control clinic or a nutritionist, for example, you may not be reimbursed—at least not without a fight.

➤ Various mechanisms discourage enrollment of high-risk patients with pre-existing conditions such as cancer. Care of people who have or have had cancer is more expensive that those who do not have the disease; therefore, insurers will try their hardest to keep you off their rolls and may use a variety of unethical and illegal tactics to do so.

Some other ways in which managed care companies oversee health care costs include the following:

➤ Requiring approval before a patient is admitted to a hospital, except in emergencies

➤ Conducting ongoing reviews of patients' treatment

➤ Day-to-day management of cases that require long-term and/or expensive care—like cancer

➤ Review of discharged hospital patients' medical records to determine the quality and necessity of all procedures and other elements of care

Physicians hate managed care. First, they can no longer get away with performing as many expensive procedures as they used to, and medical procedures are their most profitable source of income. Second, they hate having to ask permission to do what they have been trained to do. Most physicians with busy practices have had to hire people who do nothing all day long but deal with insurance companies. This is expensive.

Managed care is generally unpleasant, but it will be good for American society in the long run. Anything that brings down the cost of providing health care, but doesn't lower the quality of that care, is desirable. The problem is determining whether managed care organizations (that is, every health insurance carrier in the country) have taken so many cost-cutting steps that they have indeed jeopardized quality of care in some instances.

Appendix A

Oncology Drugs and Their Indications

*T*his section contains a list of the most commonly used drugs to treat cancer, the cancers against which they are most effective, and a "short list" of their most common side effects. Although there are many highly effective drugs still under investigation, only drugs approved by the Food and Drug Administration *(www.fda.gov)* as of the beginning of 2000 are included here. By the time you read this book, several more drugs will have been approved.

The drugs are listed by their generic names, with their trade or brand names in parentheses. The type or classification of the drugs are as follows:

AA: Alkylating agent
AB: Anti-tumor antibiotic
AM: Antimetabolite
BM: Biological response modifier
HN: Hormone or natural substance
OT: Other

Drug	Type	Cancer	Side Effects
Aldesleukin (Proleukin)	BM	Renal cell carcinoma Malignant melanoma Kaposi's sarcoma	Thrombocytopenia Nausea/vomiting Hyperbilirubinemia
Altretamine (Hexalen, Hexastat)	AA	Ovary	Leukopenia Thrombocytopenia Anemia
Amifostine (Ethyol)	OT	N/A (This drug reduces the nephrotoxicity of cisplatin in lung cancer patients	
Aminogluthethamide (Cytadre)	HN	Breast Prostate Adrenal gland	Leukopenia Nausea/vomiting Anorexia
Anastrozole (Arimidex)	HN	Breast	Leukopenia Anemia Nausea/vomiting Rash/itching Dyspnea
Asparaginase (Elspar)	OT	Leukemias Lymphomas Hodgkin's disease	Abdominal pain Nausea/vomiting Depression Itching Joint pain Dizziness Thrombocytopenia
Bacillus Calmette-Guerin (Theracys, Tice)	BM	Bladder	Anemia Leukopenia Rash
Bicalutamide (Casodex)	HN	Prostate	Anemia Nausea/vomiting Hot flashes Generalized pain
Bleomycin (Blenoxane)	AB	Squamous cell Hodgkin's disease Lymphomas Reproductive organ Testicle	Anorexia Rash/itching Fever
Busulfan (Busulflex)	AA	Myelogenous leukemia Bone marrow transplant	Myelosuppression Nausea/vomiting Hyperpigmentation Fatigue
Carboplatin (Paraplatin)	AA	Ovary Cervix Leukemias Bladder Brain	Thrombocytopenia Neutropenia Liver abnormality Nausea/vomiting Pain

Drug	Type	Cancer	Side Effects
Carmustine (BCNU)	AA	Hodgkin's disease Lymphomas Melanoma Colon/rectum Stomach	Leukopenia Thrombocytopenia Alopecia Nausea/vomiting
Chlorambucil (Leukeran)	AA	Leukemias Hodgkin's disease Lymphomas Breast Myeloma	Thrombocytopenia Leukopenia Alopecia Nausea/vomiting
Cisplatin (Platinol, Platinol-AQ)	AA	Reproductive organs Sarcomas Hodgkin's disease Lymphomas	Nausea/vomiting Hearing problems Sore throat Leukopenia Thrombocytopenia Nephrotoxicity
Cladribine (Leustatin)	OT	Hairy cell leukemia Lymphomas Hodgkin's disease	Neutropenia Myelosuppression Nausea/vomiting Rash/itching
Cyclophosphamide (Cytoxan, NEOSAR)	AA	Hodgkin's disease Lymphomas Sarcomas Leukemias	Nausea/vomiting Anorexia Neutropenia Headache Alopecia
Cytarabine (Cytosar-U, Ara-C)	AM	Leukemias Lymphomas Head and neck	Nausea/vomiting Fatigue Neutropenia Thrombocytopenia
Dacarbazine (DTIC-Dome)	AA	Hodgkin's disease Malignant melanoma Sarcomas	Nausea/vomiting Anorexia Leukopenia Thrombocytopenia
Dactinomycin (Cosmegen, Actinomycin-D)	AB	Testicle Malignant melanoma Choriocarcinoma Wilms' tumor Uterus	Nausea/vomiting Fatigue Leukopenia Thrombocytopenia
Daunorubicin (Cerubidine)	AB	Leukemias Neuroblastoma Wilms' tumor	Nausea/vomiting Leukopenia Rash Cardiotoxicity Shortness of breath
Denilleukin difitox (ONTAK)	BM	Lymphoma	Confusion Chest pain Diarrhea Weight loss Headache

Drug	Type	Cancer	Side Effects
Dexamethasone (Decadron, Hexadrol)	HN	Brain metastasis Breast Leukemias Myeloma	Nausea/vomiting Anorexia Menstrual changes Hyperglycemia
Diethylstilbesterol (DES)	HN	Prostate Breast	Nausea/vomiting Liver problems Headache Menstrual changes Impotence
Docetaxel (Taxotere, Taxol)	AB	Breast	Neutropenia Nausea/vomiting Alopecia Dyspnea
Doxorubicin (Adriamycin, Rubex)	AB	Lung Breast Bladder Ovary	Nausea/vomiting Neutropenia Mouth sores Alopecia Thrombocytopenia
Epirubicin (Ellence)	AA	Breast Leukemias Sarcomas Lymphomas Ovary	Thrombocytopenia Anemia Nausea/vomiting Alopecia Cardiotoxicity
Epoetin alpha (Epogen, Procrit)	BM	Renal failure secondary to AZT therapy in AIDS Nonmyeloid cancers	Diarrhea Fever Injection pain
Estramustin (Emcyt)	HN	Prostate Cardiotoxicity	Breast enlargement Nausea/vomiting Neutropenia
Etoposide (VePesid, VP-16)	HN	Testicle Lung Leukemias Lymphomas	Nausea/vomiting Anorexia Diarrhea Stomatitis
Filgrastim (Neupogen)	BM	Bone marrow transplant	Nausea/vomiting Infection Diarrhea
Finasteride (Proscar)	HN	Prostate	Impotence Decreased libido
Floxuridine (FUDR)	AM	Liver cancer Head and neck Breast	Nausea/vomiting Diarrhea Stomach cramps Stomatitis
Fludabarine (Fludara)	AM	Leukemias Lymphomas	Stomatitis Neutropenia Thrombocytopenia Renal toxicity

Drug	Type	Cancer	Side Effects
Fluorouracil (Adrucil, fluorouracil)	AM	Breast Stomach Liver	Nausea/vomiting Diarrhea Leukopenia Thrombocytopenia
Flutamide (Eulexin)	HN	Prostate	Nausea/vomiting Liver problems Constipation Diarrhea Bladder problems
Fluoxymestrone (Halotestin)	HN	Breast	Alopecia
Gemcitabine (Gemzar)	AM	Pancreas Lung Breast	Neutropenia Nausea/vomiting Alopecia Anemia Thrombocytopenia
Goserelin (Zoladex)	HN	Prostate	Local discomfort Dizziness Insomnia
Hydroxyurea (Hydrea, Droxia)	AM	Melanoma Ovary Cervix Prostate	Leukopenia Rash
Idarubicin (Idamycin)	AB	Leukemia	Myelosuppression Nausea/vomiting Alopecia
Ifosfamide (IFEX)	AA	Testicle Lymphomas Ovary	Bladder toxicity Alopecia Nausea/vomiting Leukopenia Thrombocytopenia
Interferon alphas (several types)	BM	Multiple myeloma Leukemias Bladder Lymphomas	Leukopenia Thrombocytopenia Nausea/vomiting Alopecia Dizziness Somnolence
Interferon beta-1B (Betaseron)	BM	Kaposi's sarcoma Renal cell carcinoma Melanoma Lung	Neutropenia Lymphopenia Nausea/vomiting Diarrhea
Interferon gamma (Actimmune)	BM	Ovary Melanoma	Leukopenia Rash Headache

Drug	Type	Cancer	Side Effects
Interleukin-3 (IL-3)	BM	Accompanies high-dose chemotherapy	Nausea/vomiting Diarrhea Fever/chills Bone pain
Irinotecan (Camptosar)	OT	Colon/rectum Lung Cervix Ovary	Neutropenia Diarrhea Nausea/vomiting Alopecia
Leucovorin calcium (Leucovorin, Wellcovorin)	OT	Osteosarcoma Head/neck Breast Lymphomas	Thrombocytosis Nausea/vomiting Diarrhea Rash/hives
Leuprolide (Lupron Depot)	HN	Prostate	Cardiotoxicity Hypertension Blood clots Hot flashes Impotence
Lomustine (CeeNu, CCNU)	AA	Hodgkin's disease Lymphomas Malignant melanoma Brain	Nausea/vomiting Neutropenia Thrombocytopenia Anorexia
Mechlorethamine (Mustargen, nitrogen mustard)	AA	Hodgkin's disease Lymphomas Lung	Nausea/vomiting Neutropenia Thrombocytopenia
Medroxyprogesterone (Provera, Depo-Provera)	HN	Endometrium Kidney	Nausea/vomiting Nervousness Insomnia Fatigue Depression
Megestrol acetate (Progestin)	HN	Breast Endometrium	Fluid retention Hot flashes Hypertension Diabetes
Melphalen (Alkeran, L-PAM)	AA	Multiple myeloma Ovary Breast	Nausea/vomiting Neutropenia Thrombocytopenia
Mercaptopurine (Purinethol, 6-MP)	AM	Leukemias	Nausea/vomiting Neutropenia Thrombocytopenia
Methotrexate (Folex, Mexate, Rheumatrex)	AM	Leukemias Sarcomas Choriocarcinoma Head and neck Lymphomas	Nausea/vomiting Diarrhea Anorexia Stomach pain
Mitomycin (Mutamycin)	AB	Colon Stomach Pancreas	Nausea/vomiting Neutropenia Thrombocytopenia Pain at IV site

Drug	Type	Cancer	Side Effects
Mitotane (Lysodren)	OT	Adrenal cortex	Anorexia Nausea/vomiting Depression Dizziness
Mitoxantrone (Novantrone)	AB	Leukemias Breast Ovary Lymphomas Prostate	Leukopenia Fatigue Nausea/vomiting Diarrhea Cardiotoxicity
Paclitaxel (Taxol)	HN	Breast Ovary Kaposi's sarcoma Lung Head/neck	Neutropenia Alopecia Stomatitis
Pentostatin (Nipent)	AM	Hairy cell leukemia	Leukopenia Lymphopenia Nausea/vomiting Diarrhea
Pipobroman (Vercyte)	AA	Leukemia	Myelosuppression Leukopenia Thrombocytopenia
Plicamycin (Mithracin)	AB	Testis	Stomatitis Thrombocytopenia Hemorrhage Alopecia Cardiotoxicity
Porfimer sodium (Photofrin)	OT	Lung	Photosensitivity Mucositis
Prednisone (Metacorten, Orasone, and others)	HN	Leukemias Hodgkin's disease Lymphomas Myeloma	Insomnia Agitation Diabetes Hypertension Ulcers Vision problems
Procarbazine (Matulane)	AA	Brain cancer	Nausea/vomiting Diarrhea Thrombocytopenia Anorexia Neutropenia
Progestins (Amen, Cycrin, Delalutin, and others)	HN	Breast Prostate Uterus Kidney	Nausea/vomiting Dizziness Headache Cardiotoxicity
Sargramostim (Leukine, Prokine)	BM	Bone marrow transplantation	Flushing Hypotension Tachycardia Anorexia Nausea/vomiting

Drug	Type	Cancer	Side Effects
Streptozocin (Zanosar)	AA	Pancreas	Nausea/vomiting Pain at IV site
Tamoxifen (Nolvadex)	HN	Breast Endometrium Ovary	Nausea/vomiting Hot flashes Headache Blurred vision Bone pain
Tegafur-uracil (UFT)	AM	Colorectal	Leukopenia Neutropenia Diarrhea
Temozolomide (Temodal)	AA	Astrocytoma	Thrombocytopenia Nausea/vomiting Convulsions Fatigue
Teniposide (Vumon)	HN	Leukemias Lung	Leukopenia Abdominal pain
Testolactone (Teslac)	HN	Breast	
Thioguanine (Tabloid)	AM	Leukemias	Nausea/vomiting Diarrhea Neutropenia Thrombocytopenia
Thiotepa (Thioplex)	AA	Breast Ovary Bladder Hodgkin's disease Lymphomas	Leukopenia Myelosuppression Stomatitis Second malignancy
Thrombopoietin (TPO)	BM	Accompanies high-dose chemotherapy	Headache
Topotecan (Hycamtin)	HN	Lung	Neutropenia Thrombocytopenia
Toremifene (Fareston)	HN	Breast	Hot flashes Nausea/vomiting
Trastuzumab (Herceptin)	BM	Breast	Chills/fever Cardiotoxicity
Tretinoin (Vesanoid)	OT	Leukemia	Leukocytosis Skin exfoliation Headache
Trimetrexate (Neutrexin)	AM	Lung Head/neck Colon	Anemia Thrombocytopenia Mucositis Leukopenia Myelosuppression

Drug	Type	Cancer	Side Effects
Tumor necrosis factor (TNF-alpha)	BM	Kaposi's sarcoma Malignant melanoma	Leukopenia Abdominal pain Nausea/vomiting
Uracil mustard (Uramustine)	AA	Leukemias Lymphomas Ovary	Myelosuppression Leukopenia Thrombocytopenia Nausea/vomiting Anorexia
Vinblastine (Velban, Velsar)	HN	Hodgkin's disease Choriocarcinoma Testis Kaposi's sarcoma	Nausea/vomiting Pain at IV site Neutropenia Alopecia
Vincristine (Oncovin, Vincasar, Vincrez)	HN	Leukemia Hodgkin's disease Neuroblastoma	Pain at IV site Constipation Alopecia Headache
Vinorelbine (Navelbine)	HN	Lung Breast	Leukopenia Neutropenia Nausea/vomiting

Drugs Used to Treat Various Cancers

All of the drugs listed in this section can be used in combination with one another.

ACTH-Producing Tumors
Aminoglutethemide
Trilostane

Acute Lymphocytic Leukemia
Asparaginase
Cyclophosphamide
Cytarabine
Dactinomycin
Daunorubicin
Dexamethasone
Doxorubicin
Etoposide
Floxuridine
Idarubicin
Ifosfamide
Mercaptopurine
Methotrexate
Mitoxantrone
Pegasparagase
Pentostatin
Prednisone
Teniposide
Thioguanine
Vincristine

Acute Nonlymphocytic Leukemia
Asparaginase
Busulfan
Cyclophosphamide
Cytabrine
Daunorubicin
Doxorubicin
Etoposide
Floxuridine

Idarubicin
Ifosfamide
Mercaptopurine
Methotrexate
Mitoxantrone
Thioguanine
Vincristine

Adrenal Cortex
Aminogluthethamide
Cisplatin
Cyclophosphamide
Dacarbazine
Doxorubicin
Etoposide
Fluorouracil
Ketoconazole
Mitotane
Streptozocin
Trilostane
Vincristine

Bladder Cancer
Adriamycin
Bacillus Calmette-
  Guerin
Bleomycin
Carboplatin
Cisplatin
Cyclophosphamide
Doxorubicin
Epirubicin
Etoposide
Floxuridine
Fluorouracil
Gallium nitrate
Gemcitabine
Ifosfamide
Interferon alphas
Methotrexate
Mitomycin
Mitoxantrone
Paclitaxel
Thiotepa
Vinblastine

Bone Lesions
Levodopa
Sodium phosphate

Brain Tumors
Busulfan
Carboplatin
Carmustine
Cisplatin
Cyclophosphamide
Dacarbacide
Dexamethasone
Etoposide
Floxuridine
Ifosfamide
Interferon
Lomustine
Mechlorethamine
Methotrexate
Prednisone
Procarbazine
Vincristine

Breast Cancer
Aminoglutethemide
Anastrozol
Carboplatin
Carmustine
Cisplatin
Chlorambucil
Cyclophosphamide
Dactinomycin
Dexamethasone
Dexrazoxane
Diethylstilbesterol
Docataxel
Doxorubicin
Epirubicin
Estradiol
Estrogens
Ethinyl
Etoposide
Floxuridine
Fluorouracil
Fluoxymesterone
Gemcitabine
Goserelin
Ifosfamide
Leucovorin calcium
Leuprolide
Lomustine
Mechlorethamine
Medroxyprogesterone
Megestrol acetate

Melphalen
Methotrexate
Methyltestosterone
Mitomycin
Mitoxantrone
Nandrolone
Pamidronate disodium
Paclitaxel
Prednisone
Progestins
Tamoxifen
Testolactone
Testosterone
Thiotepa
Toremifene
Trastuzumab
Vinblastine
Vincristine
Vinorelbine tartrate

Cervical Cancer
Altretamine
Bleomycin
Carboplatin
Cisplatin
Cyclophosphamide
Doxorubicin
Fluorouracil
Hydroxyurea
Ifosfamide
Interferon
Irinotecan
Methotrexate
Mytomycin
Procarbazine
Temozolomide
Uracil mustard
Vinblastine
Vincristine

Choriocarcinoma
Dactinomycin
Methotrexate
Vinblastine

Chronic Lymphocytic Leukemia
Asparaginase
Carboplatin
Chlorambucil
Cladibrine

Cyclophosphamide
Cytarabine
Daunorubicin
Dexamethasone
Doxorubicin
Epirubicin
Etoposide
Fludarabine phosphate
Interferon alphas
Mechlorethamine
Mercaptopurine
Methotrexate
Pentostatin
Prednisone
Sodium phosphate
Teniposide
Thioguanine
Trentinoin
Uracil mustard
Vincristine

Chronic Myelocytic Leukemia
Asparaginase
Busulfan
Cyclophosphamide
Cytabrine
Daunorubicin
Dexamethasone
Doxorubicin
Etoposide
Hydroxyurea
Interferon
Mechlorethamine
Melphalan
Mercaptopurine
Mitomycin
Mitoxantrone
Pibobroman
Prednisone
Sodium phosphate
Thioguanine
Uracil mustard
Vinblastine
Vincristine

Colorectal Cancer
Carmustine
Cyclophosphamide
Floxuridine
Fluorouracil

Interferon
Irinotecan hydrochloride
Leucovorin
Levamisol
Lomustine
Methotrexate
Mitomycin
Semustine
Streptozocin
Tegafur-uracil
Trimetrexate
Vincristine

Cutaneous T-Cell Lymphoma
Interferon
Mechlorethamine
Methotrexate
Pentostatin
Vinblastine
Vincristine

Endometrial Cancer
Altretamine
Bleomycin
Carboplatin
Cisplatin
Cyclophosphamide
Dactinomycin
Doxorubicin
Fluorouracil
Hydroxyprogesterone
Ifosfamide
Medroxyprogesterone
Megestrol acetate
Methotrexate
Tamoxifen

Esophogeal Cancer
Bleomycin
Carboplatin
Cisplatin
Doxorubicin
Fluorouracil
Methotrexate
Mitomycin
Paclitaxel
Porfimer sodium

Ewing's Sarcoma
Carmustine

Cyclophosphamide
Dactinomycin
Daunorubicin
Doxorubicin
Etoposide
Ifosfamide
Leucovorin
Vincristine

Gallbladder/Bile Duct
Floxuridine
Fluorouracil
Mitomycin

Hairy Cell Leukemia
Chlorambucil
Cladribine
Interferon
Pentostatin

Head and Neck Cancer
Bleomycin
Carboplatin
Cisplatin
Cyclophosphamide
Cytarabine
Doxorubicin
Floxuridine
Fluorouracil
Hydroxyurea
Interferon
Leucovorin calcium
Methotrexate
Mitomycin
Paclitaxel
Trimetrexate
Vinblastine
Vincristine

Hodgkin's Disease
Asparaginase
Bleomycin
Carmustine
Chlorambucil
Cisplatin
Cladribine
Cyclophosphamide
Cytabrine
Dacarbazine
Dexamethasone

Doxorubicin
Etoposide
Ifosfamide
Lomustine
Mechlorethamine
Mercaptopurine
Prednisone
Procarbazine
Streptozocin
Thiotepa
Uracil mustard
Vinblastine
Vincristine

Kaposi's Sarcoma
Aldesleukin
Bleomycin
Cisplatin
Dactinomycin
Daunorubicin
  (and liposomal)
Doxorubicin
  (and liposomal)
Etoposide
Interferon beta-1B
Paclitaxel
Tumor necrosis factor
Vinblastine
Vincristine

Kidney Cancer
Aldesleukin
Bleomycin
Cyclophosphamide
Floxuridine
Interferon beta-1B
Lomustine
Medroxyprogesterone
Methotrexate
Progestins
Vinblastine
Vincristine

Liver Cancer
Carmustine
Cisplatin
Doxorubicin
Etoposide
Floxuridine
Fluorouracil
Methotrexate

Mitoxantrone
Streptozocin

Lung Cancer (Small Cell and Non-Small Cell)
Altretamine
Amifostine
Carboplatin
Carmustine
Cisplatin
Cyclophosphamide
Doclitaxel
Doxorubicin
Etoposide
Fluorouracil
Gemcitabine
Hydroxyurea
Ifosfamide
Interferon beta-1B
Irinotecan
Leucovorin calcium
Lomustine
Mechlorethamine
Methotrexate
Mitomycin
Paclitaxel
Porfirmer sodium
Procarbazine
Teniposide
Topotecan
Trimetrexate
Uracil mustard
Vinblastine
Vincristine
Vinorelbine tartrate

Malignant Melanoma
Aldesleukin
Asparaginase
Bleomycin
Carboplatin
Carmustine
Cisplatin
Dacarbazine
Dactinomycin
Hydroxyurea
Interferon beta-1B
Interferon gamma
Lomustine
Melphalan

Procarbazine
Tamoxifen
Tumor necrosis factor
Vinblastine
Vincristine

Mesothelioma
Cisplatin

Multiple Myeloma
Carmustine
Chlorambucil
Cisplatin
Cyclophosphamide
Dexamethasone
Doxorubicin
Etoposide
Interferon alphas
Lomustine
Melphalan
Methotrexate
Pamidronate disodium
Prednisone
Procarbazine
Vincristine

Neuroblastoma
Carboplatin
Cisplatin
Cyclophosphamide
Dacarbazine
Daunorubicin
Doxorubicin
Etoposide
Ifosfamide
Teniposide
Vinblastine
Vincristine

Non-Hodgkin's Lymphoma
Altretamine
Asparaginase
Bleomycin
Carmustine
Chlorambucil
Cisplatin
Cladribine
Cyclophosphamide
Cytarabine
Daunorubicin

Denilleukin difitox
Dexamethasone
Doxorubicin
Epirubicin
Etoposide
Fludarabine phosphate
Ifosfamide
Interferon alphas
Leucovorin calcium
Lomustine
Mechlorethamine
Mercaptopurine
Methotrexate
Mitoxantrone
Prednisone
Procarbazine
Streptozocin
Teniposide
Thiotepa
Uracil mustard
Vinblastine
Vincristine

Osteosarcoma
Bleomycin
Cisplatin
Cyclophosphamide
Dactinomycin
Doxorubicin
Ifosfamide
Interferon
Leucovorin calcium
Melphalan
Methotrexate
Vincristine

Ovarian Cancer
Altretamine
Amifostine
Carboplatin
Chlorambucil
Chromic phosphate
Cisplatin
Cyclophosphamide
Dactinomycin
Docetaxel
Doxorubicin
Epirubicin
Etoposide
Floxuridine
Fluorouracil

Hydroxyurea
Ifosfamide
Interferon gamma
Irinotecan
Mechlorethamine
Melphalan
Methotrexate
Mitoxantrone
Paclitaxel
Tamoxifen
Thiotepa
Topotecan hydrochloride
Uracil mustard

Pancreatic Cancer
Cisplatin
Cyclophosphamide
Dacarbazine
Doxorubicin
Fluorouracil
Gemcitabine
Ifosfamide
Interferon
Leuprolide
Methotrexate
Mitomycin
Octreotide
Streptozocin
Trimetrexate
Vincristine

Penile Cancer
Bleomycin
Cisplatin
Methotrexate

Prostate Carcinoma
Aminoglutethemide
Bicalutamide
Buserelin
Chlorotrianisene
Chromic phosphate
Cisplatin
Cyclophosphamide
Dexamethasone
Diethylstilbesterol
Doxorubicin
Estradiol
Estramustine
Estrogens
Estrone

Ethinyl estradiol
Finasteride
Fluorouracil
Flutamide
Goserelin
Hydroxyurea
Ketoconazole
Leuprolide
Melphalan
Methotrexate
Mitomycin
Mitoxantrone
Nilutamide
Prednisone
Progestins

Reproductive Organ Cancers
Bleomycin
Cisplatin

Retinoblastoma
Carboplatin
Cyclophosphamide

Sarcomas
Cisplatin
Cyclophosphamide
Dacarbazine
Methotrexate

Skin Cancer
Bleomycin
Cisplatin
Fluorouracil
Interferon
Masoprocol
Methoxsalen

Soft Tissue Sarcoma
Asparaginase
Bleomycin
Cisplatin
Cyclophosphamide
Dacarbazine
Dactinomycin
Daunorubicin
Doxorubicin
Etoposide
Ifosfamide
Melphalan

Methotrexate
Vinblastine
Vincristine

Squamous Cell Carcinoma
Bleomycin

Stomach Cancer
Carmustine
Cisplatin
Doxorubicin
Etoposide
Fluorouracil
Leucovorin
Methotrexate
Mitomycin

Testicular Cancer
Bleomycin
Carboplatin
Chlorambucil
Cisplatin
Cyclophosphamide
Dactinomycin
Doxorubicin
Etoposide
Ifosfamide
Melphalan
Methotrexate
Nitrofurazone
Plicamycin
Vinblastine

Thyroid Cancer
Bleomycin
Cisplatin
Doxorubicin
Levothyroxine
Liothyronine
Liotrix
Melphalan
Sodium iodide
Thyroglobulin
Thyrotropin
Vincristine

Trophoblastic Neoplasms
Bleomycin
Chlorambucil

Cisplatin
Cyclophosphamide
Dactinomycin
Doxorubicin
Etoposide
Hydroxyurea
Leucovorin
Methotrexate
Vinblastine
Vincristine

Uterine Cancer
Cisplatin
Dactinomycin
Hydroxyprogesterone
Ifosfamide
Progestins

Cancer of the Vagina
Doxorubicin

Cancer of the Vulva
Bleomycin

Wilms' Tumor
Carboplatin
Cisplatin
Cyclophosphamide
Dactinomycin
Daunorubicin
Doxorubicin
Etoposide
Vincristine

Appendix B

Resources

AirLifeLine (free air transport for
  cancer patients)
6133 Freeport Boulevard
Sacramento CA 95822
(800) 446-1231

American Academy of Pain Medicine
American Pain Society
5700 Old Orchard Road
Skokie IL 60077
(708) 966-9510

American Brain Tumor Association
3725 North Talman Avenue
Chicago IL 60618
(800) 886-2282

American Cancer Society National
  Headquarters
1599 Clifton Road, N.E.
Atlanta GA 30329
(800) ACS-2345
www.cancer.org
(for state, county, and municipal
  chapters, check your phone book)

American College of Obstetricians and
  Gynecologists
409 12th Street, S.W.
Washington DC 20090
(202) 863-2528

American Dietetic Association
National Center for Nutrition and
  Dietetics
(800) 366-1655

American Institute for Cancer
  Research
1759 R Street, N.W.
Washington DC 20009
(800) 843-8114

American Pain Society
4700 West Lake Avenue
Glenville IL 60025
(847) 966-5595

American Self-Help Clearinghouse
Northwest Covenant Medical Center
25 Pocono Road
Denville NJ 07834
(800) 367-6274 (NJ only)
(201) 625-7101
www.cmhc.com/selfhelp

American Society of Clinical
  Oncology
435 North Michigan Avenue, Suite
  1717
Chicago IL 60611
(312) 644-0828

Association of Community Cancer
  Centers
11600 Nebel Street, Suite 201
Rockville MD 20852
(301) 984-9496

Biological Therapy Institute
  Foundation
P. O. Box 681700
Franklin TN 37068
(615) 790-7535

Blood and Marrow Transplant
  Newsletter
1985 Spruce Avenue
Highland Park IL 60035
(847) 831-1913
www.bmtnews.org

Bone Marrow Donors Worldwide
www.BMDW.LeidenUniv.NL

Bone Marrow Transplant Family
  Support Network
P. O. Box 845
Avon CT 06001
(800) 826-9376

Breast Cancer Advisory Center
11426 Rockville Pike, Suite 406
Rockville MD 20859
(301) 984-1020

Breast Cancer Resource Committee
1765 N Street, N.W., Suite 100
Washington DC 20036-2802
(202) 463-8040

CAN ACT (Cancer Patients Action
  Alliance) [political advocacy]
26 College Place
Brooklyn NY 11201
(718) 522-4607

Canadian Cancer Society
10 Alcorn Avenue, Suite 200
Toronto, Ontario M4V 3B1
Canada
(416) 961-7223

Cancer Care, Inc.
1180 Avenue of the Americas,
  2nd Floor
New York NY 10036
(800) 813-4673
www.cancercareinc.org

Cancer Consultation Service
237 Thompson Street
New York NY 10012
(212) 254-5031

Cancer Family Care
7162 Reading Road, Suite 1050
Cincinnati OH
(513) 731-3346

Cancer FAQ
www.cancercare.org/faq/cancer_faq.html

CancerFax
National Cancer Institute
(301) 402-5874

Cancer Guidance Hotline
1323 Forbes Avenue
Pittsburgh PA 15219
(412) 261-2211

Cancer Information Service
National Cancer Institute
Building 31, Room 10A07
Bethesda MD 20892-2580
(800) 4-CANCER
www.nci.gov

Cancer Research Foundation
  of America
1600 Duke Street, Suite 110
Alexandria VA 22314
(703) 836-4412

Cancer Research Institute
681 Fifth Avenue
New York NY
(800) 99-CANCER

Candlelighters Childhood Cancer
   Foundation
7910 Woodmont Avenue, Suite 460
Bethesda MD 20814
(800) 366-2223

Center for Mind-Body Medicine
5225 Connecticut Avenue, N.W.,
   Suite 414
Washington DC 20015
(202) 363-6632
www.healthy.net/cmbm

ChemoCare
231 North Avenue West
Westfield NJ 07090
(800) 55-CHEMO

Chemotherapy Foundation, Inc.
183 Madison Avenue
New York NY 10016
(212) 213-9292

Commonweal
   (complementary medicine)
P. O. Box 316
Bolinas CA 94924
(415) 868-0970

Coping Magazine
P. O. Box 682268
Franklin TN 37068
(615) 790-2400
copingmag@aol.com

Corporate Angel Network, Inc. (free
   air transport for cancer patients)
Westchester County Airport,
   Building 1
White Plains NY 10604
(914) 328-1313

Cure for Lymphoma Foundation
215 Lexington Avenue, 11th Floor
New York NY 10016-6023
(212) 213-9595
www.cfl.org

Families Against Cancer (FACT)
   (advocacy and support)
P. O. Box 588
Dewitt NY 13214
(315) 446-5326

Food and Drug Administration Office
   of Consumer Affairs
Room HFE-88
5600 Fishers Lane
Rockville MD 20857
(800) 532-4440

The Susan G. Komen Breast Cancer
   Foundation
5005 LBJ Freeway, Suite 370
Dallas TX 75255
(972) 855-1605

International Myeloma Foundation
2120 Stanley Hills Drive
Los Angeles CA 90046
(800) 452-2873
www.myeloma.org

Leukemia Society of America
600 Third Avenue
New York NY 10016
(800) 284-4271

Lymphoma Research Foundation
   of America
8800 Venice Boulevard, Suite 207
Los Angeles CA 90034
(310) 204-7040
www.lymphoma.org

Make Today Count (peer support)
P. O. Box 22
Osage Beach MO 65065

Medicare
U.S. Department of Health and
   Human Services
Social Security Administration
Baltimore MD 21235
(800) 772-1213

National Alliance of Breast Cancer
   Organizations
9 East 37 Street, 10th Floor
New York NY 10016
(800) 719-9154
www.nabco.org

National Association of Oncology
   Social Workers
1233 York Avenue, Suite 4P
New York NY 10021
(212) 734-8891

National Brain Tumor Foundation
785 Market Street, Suite 1600
San Francisco CA 94103
(800) 934-CURE

National Breast Cancer Coalition
1707 L Street, N.W., Suite 1060
Washington DC 20036
(800) 935-0434

National Cancer Institute
Building 31, Room 1024A
Bethesda MD 20892
(800) 422-6237
www.icic.nci.nih.gov

National Chronic Pain
   Outreach Association
7979 Old Georgetown Road,
   Suite 100
Bethesda MD 20814
(301) 652-4948

National Coalition for
   Cancer Research
426 C Street, N.E.
Washington DC 20002
(202) 544-1880

National Coalition for Cancer
   Survivorship
1010 Wayne Avenue, 5th Floor
Silver Spring MD 20910
(301) 650-8868

National Council for Reliable
   Health Information
300 East Pink Hill Road
Independence MO 64057
(816) 228-4595
www.ncrhi.org
drrenner@msn.com

National Health Information Center
P. O. Box 1133
Washington DC 20013
(800) 336-4797

National Hospice Organization
1901 North Moore Street, Suite 901
Arlington VA 22209
(800) 658-8898

National Insurance Consumer
   Organization
121 North Payne Street
Alexandria VA 22314
(703) 549-8050

National Kidney Cancer Association
1234 Sherman Avenue, Suite 200
Evanston IL 60202
(708) 332-1051
nkca@merle@acsns.nwuu.edu

National Leukemia Association
585 Stewart Avenue, Suite 536
Garden City NY 11530
(516) 222-1944

National Library of Medicine
8600 Rockville Pike
Bethesda MD 20894
(800) 638-8480
www.nlm.nih.gov

National Patient Air Transport Hotline
(800) 296-1217

National Women's Health Network
1325 G Street, N.W.
Washington DC 20005
(202) 347-1140

Ontario Cancer Information Service
755 Concession Street
Hamilton, Ontario L8V 1C4
Canada
(800) 263-6750

Patient Advocates for Advanced
   Cancer Treatment
1143 Parmelee, N.W.
Cedar Rapids MI 49504
(616) 453-1477

PDQ (Physician Data Query)
(800) 4-CANCER

People Living Through Cancer, Inc.
323 8th Street S.W.
Albuquerque NM 87102
(505) 242-3263

Reach to Recovery (for mastectomy
   patients)
American Cancer Society
(800) ACS-2345

Ronald McDonald Houses
   (for families of children
   with cancer)
National Coordinator
Golin Communications, Inc.
500 North Michigan Avenue
Chicago IL 60611
(312) 836-7384

Roxane Pain Institute
www.Roxane.com/Roxane/RPI

Skin Cancer Foundation
245 Fifth Avenue, Suite 2402
New York NY 10016
(212) 725-5176

United Cancer Council, Inc.
1803 North Meridian Street
Indianapolis IN 46202
(317) 923-6490

University of Pennsylvania Oncolink
http://cancer.med.upenn.edu/

Y-Me Breast Cancer Support Program
18220 Harwood Avenue
Homewood IL 60430
(800) 221-2141

Appendix C

Choosing an Oncologist

A Baker's Dozen of Things to Look For

➤ Make certain that he or she is board certified in oncology. *Board certification* means that a physician has undergone a course of study in a medical specialty, in this case cancer, and has passed a set of rigorous examinations in the subject. Proof of board certification will be on the physician's office wall, along with his or her other diplomas. If you don't see it (and *do* look), ask. Most people find an oncologist through referrals from friends or relatives who have had cancer, and your internist or family practitioner can give you the names of several. Also, ask yourself what's important to you in a physician: male or female, old or young, office location, office hours, personality.

➤ Try to find someone who practices at one of the major cancer centers listed in Appendix D. Not only will you get the finest medical care available at such a center, but the nurses, technicians, and other personnel are highly experienced in caring for cancer patients. If you live in a rural community far from a cancer center, you might want to think about moving temporarily to the nearest city that has one. Contact the social work department there for help in finding low-cost housing or a family who might be willing to rent you a room for the duration of your chemotherapy.

➤ Listen to the oncologist during your initial appointment. Physicians often use language you don't understand (medicalese) and won't translate unless you ask. You should not

have to ask. If you can't understand much of what the
doctor says, you might want to look elsewhere. Having
cancer and undergoing chemotherapy is stressful enough
without having a language barrier between yourself and
your oncologist.

➤ In addition to what the oncologist is actually saying, listen to
what's going on between the lines. Many physicians use the
parent-child relationship as a model for "managing" patients,
which automatically puts the patient at a disadvantage. Even
the word *manage* is patronizing and condescending. If you
feel this is going on, find another doctor. If the oncologist
doesn't listen or pay attention to what you are saying, or
doesn't make notes in your medical record about what you
say and feel, think about leaving the practice.

➤ Make certain that the oncologist will answer all your questions completely—in language that you can understand. Better
yet, he or she should be able to anticipate most of your questions. You should never be rushed through a visit or feel that
the physician is too busy to give you all the time you need.

➤ You and your oncologist should have a similar philosophy of
cancer care. That is, the two of you should expect about the
same things from the doctor-patient relationship. Don't
forget that choice is a powerful tool. *You* choose your physician and *you* choose to stay.

➤ The oncologist should see you on time—or at least as on
time as doctors ever are. Up to 15 minutes is a reasonable
time to be kept waiting. More than that is arrogant, rude,
and disrespectful.

➤ Your oncologist should always tell you why you need a certain test, procedure, or medication, as well as inform you
about their dangers and negative effects.

➤ He or she should return phone calls promptly.

➤ Your oncologist ought to make accommodations about
money: reducing the amount of the bill if you are short of
funds, or allowing you to pay off the bill a little at a time.

➤ He or she should be more than willing to oblige your request
for a second opinion. If you object to a certain treatment or
ask what the options are to a recommended treatment, you
deserve a full explanation. If the oncologist becomes defensive

or refuses to give the information you need, you have found an insecure and therefore dangerous practitioner, and you should choose someone else.

➤ If you need surgery, be sure the surgeon is board certified and is an oncologic surgeon—that is, a surgeon who has experience operating on cancer patients.

➤ You should like your doctor. You're not going to enter a marriage, but you will have a long-term relationship. Therefore serious personality conflicts will not sit well with either of you.

Appendix D

Cancer Centers

A comprehensive cancer center is a large medical center, usually part of a university teaching hospital. For complex treatment and for participation in most clinical trials, it is probably the place to be.

A *comprehensive cancer center* is a designation given by the National Cancer Institute to centers that have met rigorous criteria. A *clinical cancer center* is similar to a comprehensive one and performs many of the same functions, but it has not been so designated by the NCI. You will receive excellent care at either.

These are not the only places where you can receive chemotherapy. In fact, any competent oncologist can provide excellent cancer treatment. You also can receive excellent care at a community cancer center, which for many Americans is probably more convenient. Unless you have a very unusual disease or cannot receive the recommended treatment at a cancer center near your home, you may be better off staying in your local area for these reasons:

> ➤ Most chemotherapy is given on an outpatient basis, and when your treatment is finished for the day, it's much more pleasant—and a whole lot less expensive—to go home rather than to an impersonal hotel room.
> ➤ You will be surrounded by family, friends, and others who can support you during your illness and treatment.

> The ancillary care (nurses, technicians, and the like) at a community center is usually a lot more personal and friendly, especially if you are in your hometown. Major cancer centers tend to be impersonal, and the care is often provided with self-important hustle-bustle.

Some patients go to a comprehensive or clinical cancer center for an initial evaluation and decision about treatment regimen. Then the center discusses those decisions with a local oncologist who will actually provide the treatment. This is truly having the best of both worlds.

Comprehensive Cancer Centers (Grouped by State)

University of Alabama at
  Birmingham Comprehensive
  Cancer Center
Basic Health Sciences Building,
  Room 108
1918 University Boulevard
Birmingham AL 35294
(205) 934-6612

University of Arizona Cancer Center
1501 North Campbell Avenue
Tucson AZ 85724
(602) 626-6372

Jonsson Comprehensive Cancer
  Center
University of California at Los
  Angeles
200 Medical Plaza
Los Angeles CA 90047
(213) 206-0278

Kenneth T. Norris Jr. Comprehensive
  Cancer Center
University of Southern California
1441 Eastlake Avenue
Los Angeles CA 90033-0804
(213) 226-2370

Penrose Cancer Hospital
P. O. Box 7021
Colorado Springs CO 80933
(719) 630-5271

Yale University Comprehensive
  Cancer Center
333 Cedar Street
New Haven CT 06510
(203) 785-6338

Lombardi Cancer Research Center
Georgetown University Medical
  Center
3800 Reservoir Road, N.W.
Washington DC 20007
(202) 687-2192

Sylvester Comprehensive Cancer
  Center
University of Miami Medical School
1475 Northwest 12th Avenue
Miami FL 33136
(305) 548-4800

Johns Hopkins Oncology Center
600 North Wolfe Street
Baltimore MD 21205
(410) 955-8638

Dana-Farber Cancer Institute
44 Binney Street
Boston MA 02115
(617) 732-3214

University of Michigan Cancer Center
101 Simpson Drive
Ann Arbor MI 48109-0752
(313) 936-9583

Barbara Ann Karmanos Cancer
Institute
110 East Warren Avenue
Detroit MI 48201
(313) 745-4329

Mayo Comprehensive Cancer Center
200 First Street, S.W.
Rochester MN 55905
(507) 284-3413

Norris Cotton Cancer Center
Dartmouth-Hitchcock Medical Center
One Medical Center Drive
Lebanon NH 03756
(603) 646-5505

Albert Einstein Cancer Center
Weiler Hospital
1825 Eastchester Road
Bronx NY 10461
(212) 904-2754

Albert Einstein Cancer Center
Montefiore Medical Center
111 East 210th Street
Bronx NY 10467
(212) 920-4826

Roswell Park Cancer Institute
Elm and Carlton Streets
Buffalo NY 14263
(716) 845-4400

Columbia University Comprehensive
Cancer Center
College of Physicians and Surgeons
630 West 168th Street
New York NY 10032
(212) 305-6905

Kaplan Cancer Center
New York University Medical Center
462 First Avenue
New York NY 10016-9103
(212) 263-6485

Memorial Sloan-Kettering Cancer
Center
1275 York Avenue
New York NY 10021
(800) 525-2225

UNC Lineberger Comprehensive
Cancer Center
University of North Carolina School
of Medicine
Chapel Hill NC 27599
(919) 966-4431

Duke Comprehensive Cancer Center
P. O. Box 3814
Durham NC 27710
(919) 286-5515

Cancer Center of Wake Forest
University at the
Bowman Gray School of Medicine
300 South Hawthorne Road
Winston-Salem NC 27103
(919) 748-4354

Ohio State University Comprehensive
Cancer Center
300 West 10th Avenue
Columbus OH 43210
(614) 293-5485

Fox Chase Cancer Center
7701 Burholme Avenue
Philadelphia PA 19111
(215) 728-2570

University of Pennsylvania Cancer
Center
3400 Spruce Street
Philadelphia PA 19104
(215) 662-6364

University of Pittsburgh Cancer
Institute
200 Meyran Avenue
Pittsburgh PA 15213-2592
(800) 537-4063

The University of Texas
M.D. Anderson Cancer Center
1515 Holcombe Boulevard
Houston TX 77030
(713) 792-3245

San Antonio Cancer Institute
8122 Datapoint Drive
San Antonio TX 78229
(210) 616-5580

Vermont Regional Cancer Center
University of Vermont
1 South Prospect Street
Burlington VT 05401
(802) 656-4580

Fred Hutchinson Cancer Research
Center
1124 Columbia Street
Seattle WA 98104
(206) 667-4675

Mary Babb Randolph Cancer Center
West Virginia University
510 Medical Center Drive
Morgantown WV 26506
(304) 293-2370

The University of Wisconsin
Comprehensive Cancer Center
600 Highland Avenue
Madison WI 53792
(608) 263-8600

Clinical Cancer Centers (Grouped by State)

City of Hope National Medical Center
Beckman Research Institute
1500 East Duarte Road
Duarte CA 91010
(818) 359-8111 x 2292

University of California at Irvine
Cancer Center
101 The City Drive
Orange CA 92668
(714) 456-6310

University of California at San Diego
Cancer Center
225 Dickinson Street
San Diego CA 92103
(619) 543-6178

University of Colorado Cancer Center
4200 East 9th Avenue, Box B190
Denver CO 80262
(303) 270-7235

Robert H. Lurie Cancer Center
Northwestern University
303 East Chicago Avenue
Olson Pavilion, Room 8250
Chicago IL 60611
(312) 908-5250

University of Chicago Cancer
Research Center
5841 South Maryland Avenue,
Box 444
Chicago IL 60637
(312) 702-6180

Mayo Cancer Center
Mayo Foundation
200 First Street SW
Rochester MN 55905
(507) 284-3753

Albert Einstein College of Medicine
1300 Morris Park Avenue
Bronx NY 10461
(212) 920-4826

Kaplan Cancer Center
New York University Medical Center
550 First Avenue
New York NY 10016
(212) 263-5349

University of Rochester Cancer Center
601 Elmwood Avenue, Box 704
Rochester NY 14642
(716) 275-4911

Ireland Cancer Center
University Hospitals of Cleveland
Case Western Reserve University
2074 Abington Road
Cleveland OH 44106
(216) 844-5432

Jefferson Cancer Center
Thomas Jefferson University
233 South 10 Street
Philadelphia PA 19107
(215) 503-4645

Roger Williams Cancer Center
Brown University
825 Chalkstone Avenue
Providence RI 02908
(401) 456-2071

St. Jude Children's Research Hospital
332 North Lauderdale
Memphis TN 38105
(901) 495-3301

Vanderbilt Cancer Center
Vanderbilt University
649 Medical Research Building II
Nashville TN 37232
(615) 936-1782

Huntsman Cancer Institute
University of Utah Sciences Center
Building 533
Salt Lake City UT 84112
(801) 581-4048

Cancer Center
University of Virginia Health Sciences
   Center
Charlottesville VA 22908
(804) 924-2562

Massey Cancer Center
Medical College of Virginia
1200 East Broad Street
Richmond VA 23298
(804) 828-0450

Clinical Trials Cooperative Groups (Grouped by State)

Children's Cancer Study Group
University of Southern California
199 North Lake Avenue, 3rd Floor
Pasadena CA 91101-1859
(213) 681-3032

Brain Tumor Cooperative Group
12501 Prosperity Drive, Suite 200
Silver Spring MD 20904
(301) 680-9770

North Central Cancer Treatment
   Group
Room 75-Damon
Mayo Clinic
200 First Street, S.W.
Rochester MN 55905
(507) 284-4972

Pediatric Oncology Group
The Edward Mallinckrodt Department
   of Pediatrics
Washington University School of
   Medicine
4949 West Pine Street, Suite 2A
St. Louis MO 63108
(314) 367-3446

Cancer and Leukemia Group B
CALGB Central Office
444 Mount Support Road, Suite 2
Lebanon NH 03766
(603) 646-6333

Central Office of the Chair
444 Mount Support Road, Suite 2
Rural Route 3, Box 750
Lebanon NH 03766

Gynecologic Oncology Group
GOG Headquarters
1234 Market Street, 19th Floor
Philadelphia PA 19107
(215) 854-0770

National Wilms' Tumor Study Group
Children's Cancer Research Center
Children's Hospital of Philadelphia
3400 Civic Center Boulevard,
   9th Floor
Philadelphia PA 19104
(215) 387-5518

Radiation Therapy Oncology Group
RTOG Headquarters
American College of Radiology
1101 Market Street, 14th Floor
Philadelphia PA 19107
(215) 574-3195

National Surgical Adjuvant Project for
   Breast and Bowel Cancer
University of Pittsburgh
914 Scaife Hall, 3550 Terrace Street
Pittsburgh PA 15261
(412) 648-9720

Southwest Oncology Group
Cancer Therapy and Research Center
5430 Fredericksburg Road
San Antonio TX 78229-3533
(512) 366-9300

Intergroup Rhabdomyosarcoma Study
Department of Pediatrics
Virginia Commonwealth University
Medical College of Virginia
MCV Box 646
Richmond VA 23298
(804) 786-9602

Eastern Cooperative Oncology Group
Wisconsin Clinical Cancer Center
University of Wisconsin
Medical Science Center, Room 4725
420 North Charter Street
Madison WI 53706
(608) 263-6650

Glossary

ADENOCARCINOMA—Cancer that arises from glandular tissue

ADENOMA—Benign tumor that arises from glandular tissue

ADJUVANT CHEMOTHERAPY—Chemotherapy used along with surgery or radiation (or after an initial course of chemotherapy), usually given after all known cancer has been removed or to kill remaining metastatic cells, but sometimes given before surgery or radiation

ALKYLATING AGENTS—Cancer drugs that combine with cancer cells' DNA to prevent normal cell division

ALLOGENEIC TRANSPLANT—Transplanting tissue (in cancer, bone marrow) from one person to another

ALOPECIA—Hair loss

ALTERNATIVE MEDICINE—Treatment, often touted to cure cancer, that has not been scientifically proven or subjected to safety and efficacy testing

AMBULATORY INFUSION—Administration of chemotherapy by means of a small pump that delivers drugs slowly and gradually, minimizing side effects and allowing patients to continue their usual activities

ANALGESIC—Drug that relives pain

ANAPLASTIC—Tumor that bears no cellular relationship to the tissue in which it is growing

ANEMIA—Abnormally low hemoglobin or red blood cells

ANEUPLOID—Tumor cells that do not have the normal number of chromosomes (46), often meaning a worse prognosis

ANGIOGENESIS—Process by which new blood vessels form; in cancer, the formation of blood vessels that arise from a tumor

ANGIOGRAPHY—X-ray pictures of blood vessels taken by injecting a radio-opaque dye (contrast medium) into the vessels

ANTHRACYCLINE—Class of chemotherapeutic drugs, especially useful in lymphomas

ANTIBODY—Protein made by the body in response to a specific foreign protein (antigen)

ANTIEMETIC—Drug that prevents or minimizes nausea

ANTIGEN—Substance that activates the immune system and causes production of an antibody

ANTIMETABOLITES—Cancer drugs that bind to tumor enzymes and other chemicals and prevent tumor cell development and growth

ANTINEOPLASTIC—Drug or other substance that is used to kill abnormal cells

ASPIRATION—Removal of fluid or tissue through a needle, usually during a biopsy

ATROPHY—Withering or reduction in size of tissue, usually from lack of use

ATYPICAL—Out of the ordinary

AUTOIMMUNITY—Condition in which the body's immune system rejects its own tissues

AUTOLOGOUS TRANSPLANT—Removing a person's own bone marrow, treating it with chemotherapy, and returning it to the same person

BARIUM ENEMA—X-ray study of the large intestine taken after a contrast medium (barium) has been instilled via the rectum

BARIUM SWALLOW—X-ray study of the upper portion of the gastrointestinal tract taken after barium has been swallowed

BASAL CELL CARCINOMA—Type of skin cancer that grows very slowly

B-CELL—Lymphocyte that plays a primary role in the immune response; found in blood, lymph nodes, and various organs

BENIGN—Nonmalignant

BIOLOGIC RESPONSE MODIFIERS—Substances that have a direct anti-tumor effect, as well as an indirect one by stimulation of the immune system to fight cancer

BIOLOGICAL THERAPY—Using non-chemical substances that have a direct anti-tumor effect, or an indirect effect caused by stimulating the immune system to fight cancer

BIOPSY—Removal of tissue for examination under a microscope to detect cancer cells

BIOTHERAPY (also called biological response modifiers)—Use of biologically derived agents to help the body's immune system fight disease

BLOOD-BRAIN BARRIER—Microscopic structure in the brain that separates capillaries from nerve cells, thus preventing most substances from entering the brain; a natural protective mechanism that "backfires" when chemotherapy is attempted for brain cancer because it prevents the drug from reaching the tumor

BOLUS CHEMOTHERAPY (also called "push" chemotherapy)—Administration of chemotherapy over a short period of time, usually five minutes or less

BONE MARROW—Soft tissue located in bone cavities and composed of immature red blood cells, white blood cells, platelets, and fat

BONE MARROW SUPPRESSION—Decrease in one or more of the blood counts, often a side effect of chemotherapy or radiation

BONE SCAN—X-ray of all the bones in the body taken about two hours after injection of a radioactive tracer; shows areas of abnormality that may indicate the presence of primary tumors or metastases

BRACHYTHERAPY—Internal radiation therapy

BRAIN SCAN—X-ray of the brain taken after intravenous injection of a radioactive tracer; rarely used now because CT and MRI scans are more effective

BRONCHOSCOPY—Inspection of the bronchi (tubes leading from the trachea to the lungs) by means of a tube with a fiberoptic light attached, inserted through the mouth or nose

CACHEXIA—Wasting away due to malnutrition, usually seen in the last stages of cancer

CARCINOGENESIS—Development of cancer

CARCINOMA—Cancer that develops in the tissues covering or lining organs

CATHETER—Plastic tube that can be inserted into the body

CELL-CYCLE SPECIFIC—Chemotherapeutic drugs that kill cells only when they are dividing

CELLULAR IMMUNITY—Immunity brought about by the action of immune cells such as lymphocytes

CENTIGRAY (cGY)—Unit of measurement of radiation therapy

CERVICAL LYMPH NODES—Lymph nodes in the neck

CHEMOTHERAPY—Treatment of cancer with drugs or biologics that kill malignant cells or stop them from growing

CHROMOSOMES—Strands of genetic material that carry genes; each cell has 23 pairs

CLINICAL TRIAL—Scientific study in humans to determine benefits, side effects, and safety of a new drug or treatment

CLONE—A strain of genetically identical cells derived from a single cell

COLONY STIMULATING FACTOR—A substance that stimulates growth of bone marrow cells

COMBINATION CHEMOTHERAPY—Use of two or more anticancer drugs at the same time

COMBINED MODALITY THERAPY—Using two or more types of treatment, such as surgery and chemotherapy

COMPLETE RESPONSE—No evidence of residual cancer following treatment

CONE BIOPSY—Removal of a ring of tissue from the opening of the cervix

CONSOLIDATION—Second round of chemotherapy to further reduce the number of cancer cells

CONTROL GROUP—Participants in a randomized clinical trial who do not receive the agent being tested

COOPERATIVE GROUP—Group of physicians or cancer centers participating in the same clinical trial

CRYOPRESERVATION—Preserving tissue by storing it at a very low temperature

CRYOSURGERY—Killing tissue (e.g., cancer cells) by freezing it

CT (COMPUTERIZED TOMOGRAPHY) SCAN—Series of many x-rays taken in cross section that penetrate to a variety of depths through body tissue

CYST—Fluid-filled sac of tissue; usually benign but possibly malignant

CYTOGENETICS—Microscopic analysis of the chromosome pattern of a cell

CYTOKINE—Substance secreted by immune system cells to send messages to other immune cells; a chemical messenger

CYTOLOGY—Microscopic examination of cells

CYTOTOXIC—Poisonous to cells

DEBULKING—Removing part of a tumor to decrease its size in order to relieve symptoms or to give chemotherapy a "head start"

DNA (DEOXYRIBONUCLEIC ACID)—Basis of genetic material; passes on hereditary characteristics and information about cell growth, division, and function

DOSE LIMITING—Condition that makes it unwise to exceed a specific dose of therapeutic agent as a result of serious side effects

DOUBLE BLIND—Randomized clinical trial in which neither the participants nor the clinical investigators (physicians) know which group is receiving the agent being tested and which group is receiving the control

DRUG RESISTANCE—Development of resistance in cancer cells to a specific drug or drugs; may cause relapse of a patient in remission despite continued therapy with those drugs

DYSPLASIA—Abnormal development or changes in cells that may become malignant

EDEMA—Accumulation of fluid within tissues

ELECTROLYTES—Chemicals (e.g., sodium, potassium, and chloride,) found in tissues and blood

ELECTROMAGNETIC FIELD—Combination of electric and magnetic fields that radiate from electric cables, power lines, and some electrical appliances and fixtures

ELECTRON BEAM RADIATION—External radiation therapy

ENDOCRINE GLAND—Gland that secretes a hormone, such as the thyroid, ovary, and pituitary

ENDOSCOPE—Instrument designed to see into hollow organs or body cavities; usually has a fiberoptic light attached

ENDOSCOPY—Examination of hollow organs or body cavities with an endoscope

ENZYMES—Proteins that play a role in specific chemical reactions

EPIDURAL—Space surrounding the spinal cord into which catheters can be placed for anesthesia or analgesia

EPITHELIAL TISSUE—Skin

ESTROGENS—Group of female sex hormones

EXCISION—Surgical removal of tissue

EXTRAVASATION—Leakage into the surrounding tissue of intravenous fluids, especially chemotherapeutic agents

FIBEROPTICS—Flexible tubes that transmit light by means of glass fibers

FINE NEEDLE ASPIRATION—Insertion of a small needle into a tumor to withdraw a sample of tissue for microscopic examination

FIRST-LINE THERAPY—The first drug or combination used to treat cancer

GAMMA GLOBULIN—Proteins in the blood that contain antibodies

GENE—Unit of DNA capable of transmitting a single characteristic from parent to offspring

GRAFT-VERSUS-HOST DISEASE—Condition after bone marrow transplantation in which grafted (donated) tissue may recognize the tissue of the host (patient) as foreign and try to destroy it

GRANULOCYTE (NEUTROPHIL)—Most common type of white blood cell; kills bacteria

HEMATOCRIT—Measure of red blood cell content of whole blood

HEMATOLOGIST—Physician who specializes in blood diseases

HEMATOPOIETIC—Pertaining to blood-forming organs such as bone marrow

HEMOGLOBIN—Measure of the oxygen-carrying capacity of red blood cells

HEPATIC—Pertaining to the liver

HISTOLOGY—Appearance of tissue under the microscope

HORMONAL ANTICANCER THERAPY—A type of therapy that takes advantage of some cancers' tendency to stabilize or shrink if certain hormones are administered

HORMONES—Substances released by the endocrine glands that control growth, metabolism, reproduction, and other body functions

HUMANIZED ANTIBODY—Laboratory-produced antibody that is predominantly human but contains minute mouse portions to minimize rejection by the immune system

HUMORAL IMMUNITY—Immunity mediated by substances such as proteins (gamma globulin) produced by the immune system

HYPERPLASIA—Overgrowth of normal cells; not a precursor of cancer

HYPERTHERMIA—Increased body temperature; can be used to kill cancer cells

IMMUNE SYSTEM—Mechanism that resists and fights disease; composed of white blood cells and antibodies, which react to the presence of foreign substances

IMMUNITY—A state of defense against infections or foreign substances

IMMUNOSUPPRESSION (IMMUNODEFICIENCY)—Having decreased immunity

IMMUNOTHERAPY—Use of biological agents to stimulate the immune system to attack cancer cells

INDUCTION—Initial course of chemotherapy

INFLAMMATION—Triggering of body defenses causing white cells to pour into tissues, characterized by heat, pain, and swelling

INFUSION—Slow intravenous delivery of a drug

IN SITU—Earliest stage of cancer when the tumor is still confined to the place where it originally developed

INTERFERONS—Substances produced in response to infection; can be artificially manufactured by recombinant DNA technology

INTERLEUKINS—A group of cytokines that convey molecular messages between cells of the immune system

INTRAMUSCULAR —Injection of a drug into the muscle

INTRAPERITONEAL—Delivery of drugs and fluids into the abdominal cavity

INTRATHECAL—Administration of drugs into the spinal fluid

INTRAVENOUS—Administration of drugs into a vein

INVASIVE CANCER—Cancer that spreads to adjoining healthy tissue from its original site

INVESTIGATIONAL DRUG—Drug that is still being tested in humans prior to licensure by the Food and Drug Administration

LAPAROTOMY—Surgical incision into the abdomen

LAPAROSCOPY—Insertion into the abdomen of a laparoscope, with a fiberoptic bundle attached to visualize abdominal contents

LASER—A highly concentrated beam of light that can vaporize tissue, used like a surgical instrument

LEUKOCYTE—White blood cell

LEUKOCYTOSIS—Increase in the number of leukocytes in the blood

LEUKOPENIA—Decrease in the number of leukocytes in the blood

LINEAR ACCELERATOR—Machine that produces high-energy beam radiation

LOCALIZED—Cancer confined to the site of origin without evidence of spread

LUMBAR PUNCTURE—Removal of spinal fluid for examination under a microscope

LUMPECTOMY—Surgical removal of a tumor from the breast

LYMPH NODES—Small, oval-shaped organs located throughout the body that contain clusters of lymphocytes to filter out and destroy bacteria, foreign substances, and cancer cells; connected to one another by small vessels called lymphatics

LYMPH SYSTEM—The system of lymph nodes and lymphatics

LYMPHOCYTE—White blood cells that produce antibodies and destroy invading organisms and cancer cells

LYMPHOKINE—A cytokine secreted by lymphocytes

LYMPHOMA—Cancer(s) that originate in the lymphatic system

MACROPHAGE—White blood cell that ingests and destroys invading organisms

MALIGNANT—Cancerous

MARGIN—Healthy tissue surrounding a tumor that is removed with the tumor during surgery to provide a safety zone

MEDIAN DURATION OF RESPONSE—The median length of time that a group of patients (usually investigational drug subjects) responds to therapy

MELANOMA—A particularly virulent type of skin cancer

METABOLISM—The sum of all chemical changes occurring in tissue (e.g., the way nutrients in foods are used by the body or the way drugs are broken down by the body)

METASTASIS—Spread of cancer from the original site to another part of the body

MILLIGRAMS/METER SQUARED (mg/m^2)—Formula to calculate dosage of chemotherapy drugs based on surface area of the body

MITOSIS—Cell reproduction or division

MONOCLONAL ANTIBODY—Antibody, manufactured by genetic engineering, that reacts to a specific antigen or is directed against a specific type of cancer

MRI (MAGNETIC RESONANCE IMAGING)—Creation of body images through the interaction of a magnetic field and radio waves; used to diagnose cancer and other diseases

MUCOSA (MUCOUS MEMBRANE)—Inner lining of the gastrointestinal tract, including mouth and throat, as well as other tissues such as the vagina

MUCOSITIS—Inflammation of mucous membranes, often a side effect of chemotherapy

MULTIMODALITY—Combination of two or more types of treatment

MYELOBLATION—Killing bone marrow with radiation or chemotherapy

MYELOMA—Cancer that arises in plasma cells of bone marrow

MYELOSUPPRESSION—Fall in blood counts caused by chemotherapy

NADIR—The lowest point of blood cell production

NARCOTICS—Analgesic drugs that are very effective for relief of cancer pain

NATIONAL CANCER INSTITUTE—Part of the National Institutes of Health, a federal agency located in Bethesda, Maryland, which does cancer research, supervises clinical trials of cancer treatment, and provides information to the public about all aspects of cancer

NECROSIS—Disintegration or death of tissue; what happens to cancer cells after exposure to chemotherapy

NEEDLE BIOPSY—Removing a small amount of tissue by inserting a needle into a tumor

NEOADJUVANT CHEMOTHERAPY—Chemotherapy given before surgery or radiation

NEOPLASM—New abnormal growth that may be benign or malignant

NERVE BLOCK—Temporarily or permanently numbing a nerve to alleviate pain

NEUROTOXICITY—Malfunction of a nerve, sometimes a side effect of chemotherapy

NEUTROPENIA—Abnormally low number of neutrophils, a common side effect of some chemotherapeutic drugs

NEUTROPHIL (GRANULOCYTE)—Type of white blood cell that fights infection

NODULE—Small lump or tumor that may be benign or malignant

NONCELL-CYCLE SPECIFIC—Chemotherapeutic drugs that destroy cells that are not actively dividing

ONCOGENE—DNA within a certain gene that, when activated by one of many stimuli, contributes to the transformation of normal cells into malignant ones

ONCOLOGIST—Physician who specializes in the treatment of cancer

ONCOLOGY—Medical specialty dealing with cancer

PALLIATIVE—Treatment that aims to improve quality of life but is not expected to be curative

PARTIAL RESPONSE—Fifty percent or greater (but less than 100 percent) reduction in tumor size

PATHOLOGIST— Physician who specializes in examining cells and tissues

PATHOLOGY—Study of disease through examination of tissues, organs, and other materials

PERFORMANCE STATUS—Measure of how well a cancer patient is functioning; also known as Karnofsky score

PERIPHERAL BLOOD STEM CELLS—Stem cells derived from peripheral blood rather than bone marrow

PET (POSITRON EMISSION TOMOGRAPHY)—Scan that detects abnormal growth rate of cells

PHOTODYNAMIC THERAPY—Injection of a light-sensitizing chemical, followed by application of light in order to enhance laser therapy and other cancer treatments

PLACEBO—Inert substance (commonly called a "sugar pill," although it is not made of sugar) used in some clinical trials and given to participants not receiving the active substance under investigation; never used in cancer clinical trials

PLATELET—Cell that circulates in the blood; responsible for the initial stage of the clotting mechanism

POLYCYTHEMIA—Excessively high red blood cell count

POLYP—Growth that protrudes from mucous membranes; may eventually become malignant

PORT—Disk with a soft center that is surgically implanted under the skin, connected to a large vein via a small catheter; drugs injected into the port find their way into the circulatory system without subjecting the patient to repeated venipuncture

PRIMARY TUMOR—Original cancer tumor

PROGNOSIS—Likely outcome of a disease in an individual

PROGRESSION—Growth or advancement of cancer; worsening of the disease

PROPHYLAXIS—Prevention

PROSTATE SPECIFIC ANTIGEN (PSA)—Substance derived from the prostate gland whose elevation may indicate the presence of cancer; a tumor marker

PROTOCOL—Detailed written description of a cancer treatment program or clinical trial

RADICAL SURGERY—Extensive surgery to remove tumor as well as adjacent structures and lymph nodes

RADIOISOTOPE—Element that emits energy from its nucleus and can be attached to a monoclonal antibody to deliver radiation to cancer cells

RADIOLOGIST—Physician specializing in x-rays and other radiation and imaging techniques

RADIOTHERAPY (RADIATION THERAPY)—Use of radiation to treat cancer by killing cells

RANDOMIZATION—Act of randomly (by chance) dividing participants in a clinical trial into halves or thirds, one group of which receives the agent being tested

RECEPTOR—Specific protein within a cell or on its surface that, when activated by specific substances such as hormones and drugs, triggers biological responses in the cell

RECURRENCE—Reappearance of cancer after therapy has put it into remission

RED BLOOD CELL—Cell that brings oxygen to tissues and removes carbon dioxide

REFRACTORY—Used to describe tumors that do not respond to chemotherapy

REGIONAL INVOLVEMENT—Spread of cancer from its original site to nearby surrounding tissue

REGRESSION—Shrinkage of a tumor as a result of therapy

RELAPSE—Reappearance of cancer after it has been treated

REMISSION—Partial or complete shrinkage of cancer as a result of therapy; period when the disease is under control

RESECTION—Surgical removal of tissue

RESISTANCE—Failure of a tumor to respond to therapy

RNA (RIBONUCLEIC ACID)—Nucleic acid present in all cells and similar to DNA; the biochemical blueprint for formation of protein by cells

SALVAGE—Attempt to cure a patient by second-line or third-line therapy after first-line treatment has failed

SARCOMA—Cancer arising from bone, muscle, connective, or other supporting tissue

SECOND-LINE TREATMENT—Chemotherapy used in patients who did not respond well to first-line therapy

SECOND-LOOK SURGERY—Operation to determine the effectiveness of initial therapy or to discover residual or recurrent cancer

SEPSIS (SEPTICEMIA, BACTEREMIA) — Bacterial growth in the bloodstream

SQUAMOUS CELL CARCINOMA—Cancer arising from the skin or surfaces of structures such as the mouth, cervix, or lungs

STAGING—Process of determining how far cancer has spread; determines course of treatment and prognosis

STANDARD TREATMENT—Cancer treatment that has been generally accepted by oncologists as appropriate and effective for a particular cancer, and that has been approved by the Food and Drug Administration as safe and effective for that cancer

STATISTICAL SIGNIFICANCE—The likelihood that a given result did not occur by chance

STEM CELLS—Progenitor cells that grow and differentiate to develop into red and white blood cells and platelets

STEROIDS—Fat-soluble chemicals, including cortisone and some hormones, essential for many physiologic functions; some derivatives used in cancer therapy

STOMATITIS—Inflammation or soreness of the mouth, a common side effect of chemotherapy

SYSTEMIC DISEASE—Disease that involves the entire body rather than a localized site

THROMBOCYTOPENIA—Abnormally low number of platelets

THROMBOSIS—Formation of a blood clot

TIME TO PROGRESSION—The length of time between initiation of treatment and reappearance of a tumor

TISSUE—Collection of cells of the same type

TOXIC REACTION—Particularly severe side effect

TUMOR—Lump, mass, or swelling; may be either benign or malignant; the central malignant source of a cancer

TUMOR MARKER—Chemical in the blood produced by certain cancers; measuring them is useful for diagnosis and treatment

TUMOR NECROSIS FACTOR—Natural protein produced by the body that may cause tumors to shrink

ULTRASOUND—High-frequency sound waves used to create an image of structures inside the body

UNDIFFERENTIATED—Tumor that looks "wild" under the microscope (doesn't resemble the tissue of origin); these tend to grow and spread faster than well-differentiated tumors

VENIPUNCTURE—Inserting a needle into a vein

VIRUS—Unicellular infectious agent that invades cells, alters their chemistry, and causes them to produce more viruses; several viruses are known to cause cancer in animals

WELL-DIFFERENTIATED TUMOR—Tumor whose cells resemble the normal tissue from which it originated

WHITE BLOOD CELLS—Cells that fight infection

Index

B

B-lymphocytes (B-cells), 40, 45, 46
Bacillus Calmette-Geurin (BCG), 46–47, 55
Bacteria, 11
Basal cell carcinoma, 6, 145
Basophils, 40, 45
Bee pollen, 196
Bile duct surgery, 136
Biochemical approach, to combination chemotherapy, 28
Biofeedback, 164
Biological markers. *See* Tumor markers
Biological response modifiers. *See* Agents, for biological therapy
Biological therapy, 43–44, 56–57
  agents used in, 44, 52–56
  genetics and, 43, 47–49
  immune system and, 44–47
  side effects of, 85–86
  types of, 49–52
Biopsy, 16, 38, 125
Bladder
  inflammation of, 120–121
  surgery on, 136–137
  toxicity of, 106–107
Blood
  banking before surgery, 126
  components of, 38–41
  function of, 37
  metastasis through, 16
  tumor markers in, 41–42
Blood flukes, 11
Blood growth factors, 52–54, 63–64, 89–90
Bone cancer
  pain and, 151
  surgery for, 137–138
  types of, 7
Bone marrow, 38
Bone marrow transplantation (BMT), 59–61
  complications of, 66–68
  decisions about, 64–65
  future of, 68–69

high-dose chemotherapy and, 30
monoclonal antibodies and, 50
procedure for, 65–66
types of, 61–64
Bowels
  obstructions of, 121
  surgery on, 139–140, 146
Brain cancer
  radiation therapy for, 116
  surgery for, 138
  types of, 9
Breast cancer, 5
  behavior and, 13
  clinic prevention trial and, 74–76
  combination chemotherapy and, 28
  HER-2 treatment for, 44, 50–51
  surgery for, 138–139
Breast Cancer Prevention Trial (BCPT), 74–76
Breathing difficulty, as side effect, 67, 107, 121

C

Cachexia, 97
Cancer
  causes of, 10–15
  demographics of, 1–2
  list of drugs for specific, 220–224
  tests for, 19
Cancer centers, 235–236
  list of, 236–240
Carbohydrates, 166–167
Carcinogens
  demographics and, 1
  genetics and, 10
  list of suspected, 15
  in workplace, 14–15
Carcinoma of unknown primary (CUP), 9
Carcinomas, 5–7
Cardiac toxicity, 108
Cataracts, 66
Central nervous system

Dose-limiting toxicity, 28
Droperidol, 94–95
Drugs, for chemotherapy, 24–27
  administration of, 33–36
  dosage for, 33
  duration of treatment with, 36
  lists of, 211–224
  manufacture/approval/control
    of, 76–80
  resistance to, 29–30
  see also Agents, for biological
    therapy
Drugs, for pain relief, 156–157
  addiction and, 153, 160–161
  adjuvant, 161
  side effects of, 158–160
  types of, 157–158
Dysplasia, 3

E
Electromagnetic fields (EMFs),
  13–14
Empirical approach, to
  combination chemotherapy, 29
Endocrine drugs, 26–27
Endoscopic surgery, 132
Endostatin, 57
Eosinophils, 39, 45
Epstein-Barr virus, 8, 12
Erythropoietin (EPO), 39, 53
Esophagus, surgery on, 140
Estrogen, 5
Ewing's sarcoma, 7
Exercise, 164
Extravasation, 153

F
Family. See Genetics
Fat, 167–168
Fatigue
  lack of appetite and, 178–180
  as side effect, 67, 86–88, 119
  as symptom, 18
FDA (Food and Drug
  Administration)

acupuncture and, 191
dietary supplements and, 194
drug approval and, 76–80
web site of, 193
Febrile neuropenia, 54
Fee-for-service insurance, 202
Feline leukemia virus (FeLV), 12
Fever, as symptom, 18
Fiber, 167
Flukes, 11
Folkman, Judah, 56–57
Fungi, 11

G
Gallbladder surgery, 140
Gastrointestinal toxicity,
  92–103
  anorexia, 97–99
  constipation, 102–103
  diarrhea, 100–101
  nausea/vomiting, 92–97
  stomatitis, 99–100
Gender, 1–2
Gene p53, 48, 51
Gene therapy, 51–52. See also
  Genetics
Genentech, Inc., 50
Genetics, 2, 10–11
  biological therapy and, 43,
    47–49
  breast cancer and, 5
  see also Gene therapy
Gerson diet/treatment, 197
Gliomas, 9
Gonadal toxicity, 109–111
Gordon, James S., 187
Graft rejection, 68
Graft versus host disease
  (GVHD), 68
Granisetron, 95
Granulocyte colony-stimulating
  factor, 55
Guided imagery, 163

K

Kaposi's sarcoma, 7, 137
Kelly metabolic therapy, 197–198
Kidneys
    function of, 106
    surgery on, 141

L

L-aspariginase, 26
Lactose intolerance, 178
Laser treatment, 131–132
Leatrile, 198–199
Lesions, 3
Leukemias, 7–9
Leukopenia, 88–91
Li-Fraumeni syndrome, 2
Liver
    disease of, 67
    surgery for, 141–142
Livingston-Wheeler therapy, 200
Lorazepam, 94
Lumbar puncture, 35
Lung cancer, 10
    gender and, 2
    surgery for, 142
    types of, 142
Lymphatic system, 16
Lymphocytes, 40
Lymphokines, 45
Lymphomas, 7–9
Lymphosarcomas, 7–9

M

Macrobiotic diet, 198
Macrophages, 54–55
Malignancy, 2–3. *See also* Tumors
Malignant melanoma, 5
    surgery for, 145–146
    vaccine therapy for, 46–47
Managed care, 206–209
Manner metabolic cancer
    therapy, 198
Marijuana, 95
Massage, 163, 192, 196

Mastectomy, 138–139
Medicaid, 203–204, 207
Medicare, 203, 207
Medigap insurance, 203
Melanoma. *See* Malignant
    melanoma
Melanoma-associated antigens
    (MAAs), 46–47
Meningioma, 9
Menopause, 111
Metastases, 4, 16–17
Metoclopramide, 95
Microbial diet, 90
Microphages, 44
Minerals, 168–169
Mitotic inhibitors, 26
Monoclonal antibodies (MAbs)
    diagnosis with, 50
    treatment with, 50–51
Monocytes, 40
MOPP therapy, 28
Mouth
    dryness of, 177
    sores in, 176
Mucositis, 97, 99, 176–177
Multiple myeloma, 9
Music, 163
Mutation, of genes, 10–11

N

Narcotics, 159–160
National Surgical Adjuvant Breast
    and Bowel Project, 74
    contact information for, 76
Naturopathy, 192
Nausea, 92–97, 175–176
Neck surgery, 141
Neoplasms, 3
Nerve block, 129, 162
Neumega, 55
Neuroablation, 161
Neuroblastoma, 9
Neurological toxicity, 108–109
Neutropenia, 52, 88–91
Neutrophils, 39, 45, 54–55

New England Journal of Medicine,
181–182, 183
Nitrosamines, 11
Non-Hodgkin's lymphoma, 8
Nongliomas, 9
Nonmedical pain relief, 163–164
Nontraditional therapy, 181–183
complementary to mainstream
therapy, 181, 187–193
guidelines/warnings about,
184–186
harmful, 194–195
trends in, 183–184
unproven, 196–200
useless, 196
Nosocomial infection, 131
NSAIDS, 159
Nutrition
basics of, 165–169
chemotherapy and, 169–172
nontraditional therapies and,
190–191
ways to maintain good,
171–180

O

Occult primary source, 9
Off-label drug use, 79–80
-oma, 3
Ommaya reservoir, 35
Oncogenes, 10, 43
Oncologist
decisions by, about
chemotherapy, 23, 32
questions for, about
chemotherapy, 22–23
for radiation, 118
reporting side effects to, 83–85,
89, 109
tips for choosing, 231–233
Ondansetron, 95
Opoids, 157–158
Oral administration, of drugs,
33, 34
Osteosarcoma, 7
Ovarian cancer, 6–7

behavior and, 13
surgery for, 142
Oxygen therapy, 199–200

P

Pain
assessing/describing, 154–156
changing attitudes toward,
149–150
methods to control, 156–163
misconceptions about, 153–154
nontraditional therapies for,
163–164, 191–192
reasons cancer causes, 150–152
as symptom, 18
from treatments, 152–153
types of, 155
Pancreatic cancer, 6
surgery for, 142–143
Patient-controlled analgesia (PCA),
129–130
Patient, role of, in treatment,
186–187
Penis, surgery on, 143
Periosteal sarcoma, 7
Peripheral neuropathy, 153
Peripheral stem cell
transplantation, 63–64, 65
Peripheral venous access, for
drugs, 34
Perphenazine, 94
Pets, benefits of, 164
Pharmaceuticals. *See* Drugs
Photodynamic laser therapy, 132
Physician. *See* Oncologist
Physicians Data Query (PDQ), 80
PICC line, 34
Pituitary gland, surgery on, 143
Plant alkaloids, 26, 30
Plasma, 38, 41
Plasma cell neoplasms, 9
Platelets, 40–41, 53
Pneumonia, 67
Polymorphonuclear leukocytes, 45
Prayer, 163